Praise

"Ravi Sahay has simplified and distilled the ancient science of Ayurveda to practical and usable tips for the modern man. His book is replete with easy-to-apply tips you can experiment with and incorporate into your daily life resulting in a meaningful and positive impact on your well-being. Ravi has translated learnings from his journey to wellness into an excellent resource for everyone."

— Suresh Ramaswamy,
author of *Just Be: Transform Your Life and Live as Infinity*

"Ravi Sahay's new book, *May You BE Healthy*, is a compendium of health and wellness advice that seeks to combine the ancient healing techniques of Ayurveda with the recently discovered knowledge of applied physiology of the West. A daunting task, which he tackles with skill and wisdom. The result is a practical handbook of East-West lifestyle medicine, complete with exercises, meditations and recipes, a worthy addition to everyone's library."

— Tom Dwyer, M.D.

"Ravi's research regarding chronic inflammation, stress, and the role of the microbiome on overall health is not only poignant, but very relevant."

— Gregory Carlson, D.D.S

"Some people write books, but this one was written by a soul, a soul with his hand extended, wanting and willing and quite capably able to lead those who seek higher levels of health to do so. As I read the book I thought, this guy is a cartographer. Never have I seen such a detailed, bullet pointed, organized map to help the health compromised seeker to find their way back to health."

— Scott Walker, DC,
Founder of Neuro Emotional Technique &
Founder of ONE Research Foundation

"This book beautifully describes the personal experience of various chronic ailments, which is mainly due to inflammation and how to deal with them with lifestyle changes—very valuable for us all."

— Bharat B. Aggarwal, Ph.D. Director,
Inflammation Research Center, San Diego, California; USA

"I recommend this book for anyone seeking to live a more well-balanced lifestyle. Packed with practical tips and ancient wisdom, you'll learn simple strategies you can put into place immediately to begin to reverse health issues and live a more vibrant, holistic life."

— Cindy Blaser,
Functional Diagnostic Nutrition Practitioner

"In *May You BE Healthy*, Mr. Sahay lays the foundation for preventing disease and living a life of health and wellness. He shares his journey of healing and educates us on the traditional health practices of Ayurveda combined with current research to promote health and healing."

— Michael Stubblefield, L.Ac

"This book is an unique prescription to BE healthy using the ancient wisdom of holistic medicine and modern discovery of Microbiome and anti-inflammatory living. Ravi's book leads us by his own example and powerfully empowers us towards this goal of health and vitality, which is our birthright."

— Dr. Lobsang Dhondup,
Traditional Tibetan Medicine

"Both Christopher Columbus and Marco Polo were ahead of their time seeking the riches of India. Now, Ravi has brought the riches of the rishis from our beloved India to the forefront of our health crisis. Coincidence? Very unlikely! Serendipity of this magnitude defies credibility. This compelling read brings to mind how our younger generations can easily promote prevention of chronic disease issues."

— Miguel Watley, DC

"Ravi is a self-learned man, highly-educated, a practitioner of yoga, and a supporter of the Self-Realization Fellowship. He has devoted the last 20 years of his life in educating himself studying Indian Ayurvedic medicine to the application of self-care to the modern man. Please read his story. You are in for a pleasant surprise on how much clarity he has provided to taking self-care of the basic health issues for your life."

— Manjula Jain,
Online Cooking Teacher

"In simple, straightforward language, Ravi provides wisdom that has been tested by the annals of time, tested by modern medicine, and tested via his own lived experience. I have read this book thoroughly and it is helping me each day. And it will help you, too. And you don't have to do everything to get benefits. Even doing what you can, when you can, to the best you can will start you down a road to true well-being!"

— John T. Salatti, J.D., M.Div.

May You BE Healthy

Well-being
for Pennies a Day

Ravi Sahay

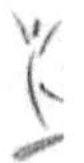

Projectwellbeing.org
San Diego, California, USA

May You BE Healthy: Well-being for Pennies a Day
Ravi Sahay

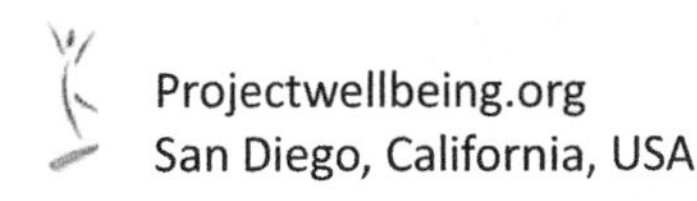

Projectwellbeing.org
San Diego, California, USA

For more information, email: ravi.sahay@gmail.com

ISBN: # 978-1-7359360-0-0 (Paperback)
ISBN: # 978-1-7359360-1-7 (eBook)

Printed in the United States of America

Cover design: Prasun Kumar
Page design: Amit Dey
Book concept: Amitabh Divakar

Concept Designer's statement: Our health is governed by three internal forces: ojas, tejas, and prana, the potential vitality, intensity, and force we experience as life. The cover depicts these three aspects of nature. The blooming of the lotus and the mudra depict a harmonious, benevolent transformation. In traditional wisdom, it is a blessing of good health.

In loving memory of the rishis of India for their
gift of Ayurveda, the science of longevity
and well-being for all.

For my beloved sister, Vidya didi, and
my dear brother, Bharatji, who
motivated me to persevere and experience
Ayurvedic healing.

Sarve Sukhinah Santu
May all be happy.

Contents

Foreword

After his heart attack in 2003, Ravi Sahay read Dr. Dean Ornish's Program for reversing heart disease and ultimately participated in the Healing Hearts program where I served as medical director at Scripps Hospital in La Jolla California. By the time I met Ravi, he had documented coronary artery disease and a left anterior descending artery stent. As an interventional cardiologist I soon realized that stents were effective only as an acute treatment for vascular disease but did nothing to reverse the underlying cause.

After reading my first book, *The Heart Speaks*, Ravi became more aware of the stress in his life and the impact stress was having on his health. He continued to struggle with hypertension and later developed cardiomyopathy and congestive heart failure. He realized inflammation was the root cause for many of his health challenges prompting him to pursue aggressive lifestyle change. His chronic inflammatory conditions had spanned beyond his heart and included eczema and sinusitis. Both stress and chronic gum disease were additional inflammation triggers. With an earnest desire to heal, Ravi persevered with my treatment recommendations and made many lifestyle changes including a healthier eating pattern, increased exercise, daily detoxification, and stress reduction.

Ravi is not a typical patient; he is an empowered one. In 2006, he wrote a book, *My Health is Your Wealth*, about his conviction that inflammation is the smoking gun for most chronic diseases. In that book, Ravi hypothesized that Candida overgrowth and/or Ayurveda Dosha imbalance are the possible root causes of many chronic conditions. Ravi started to experiment with lifestyle changes including diet, exercise, daily nasal irrigation, and other detoxification practices, including natural antifungals.

Ravi realized early on, that gut health and brain health are closely connected. He learned that immunity is the result of a dynamic balance of the complex ecosystem inside our body—our microbiome. Medical advances in understanding the microbiome has brought new knowledge and hope to understanding and treating chronic disease.

May You BE Healthy, provides a detailed and well-constructed map for building a strong immune system naturally. Ravi's book combines the ancient wisdom of Ayurveda with modern knowledge of the Microbiome and provides practical tips for a healthy life.

As we know, food is medicine. Ravi provides practical information on nutrition and explains what prebiotic and probiotic foods are, and how they are essential for a healthy microbiome. In addition, Ravi provides a delicious and nourishing array of recipes that are anti-inflammatory and promote a healthy gut microbiome.

Ravi thoughtfully discusses the ways in which our personal choices can affect our health, something I consistently discuss with my patients. Our lifestyle affects our energy, clarity of thinking, ability to fight off illness and is linked to every chronic disease. Ravi highlights how we all need to strive for balance; physically, emotionally, mentally and spiritually. This mind-body-spirit way of living enhances health and well-being.

Like many physicians and healthcare providers, I was trained to treat disease after it occurs. I have dedicated the last 20 years of my life retraining myself and others to think differently about the creation of health. My goal is to serve as a catalyst for change by empowering individuals to transform their life and by empowering healthcare providers to prevent disease utilizing the wisdom of all global healing traditions.

Ravi is one of those empowered patients and this book is a do-it-yourself manual for well-being. I sincerely hope this book will accelerate the healing you wish to see in your life.

Many Blessings for health and healing,

Mimi Guarneri, MD, FACC, ABIHM
President, Academy of Integrative Health and Medicine

Introduction

May You BE Healthy is meant for the well-being of all. "BE" connotes "Being" as in "Well-being," our natural state. Our body is a marvelous organism that changes dynamically and ideally to seek balance all the time, what scientists define as homeostasis. The dictionary meaning is the tendency toward a relatively stable equilibrium between interdependent elements, especially as maintained by physiological processes.

Well-being combines the state of happiness and health where we are free from all dis-ease, physical, mental, emotional, or social. This state of well-being can be achieved by all—rich and poor alike—hence the subtitle: *Well-being for Pennies a Day.*

I hope that reading about my journey from chronic diseases to well-being will inspire and motivate you. I humbly share the lessons in this book. In taking charge of our own health, we will also be able to lessen the looming healthcare crisis in this country.

My Story

In 2003, at the age of 55, I had a heart attack. All at once, life slowed down and I changed course. I made the most important decision of my life—I entrusted a pioneer integrative cardiologist who steered me through my various heart ailments to complete wellness today.

As a heart patient, I became proactive about lifestyle and diet changes. For a while, my health showed improvement. However, the changes I initially made were not enough. In 2007, I was diagnosed with congestive heart failure. Then in 2012, I experienced acute breathlessness that required an emergency room visit and hospitalization. Though my heart recovered within three days in acute care and my heart ejection fraction—the total amount of blood pumped out with each heartbeat—improved to the mid-30s, the doctors decided to implant a pacemaker/defibrillator (AICD) to bring it up to the normal range of 55-75.

As I look back, I realize that it was not one disease or major illness that caused my health issues. Instead, it was a gradual degradation of well-being owing to the low chronic inflammation that worsened as I reached mid-life. I discovered that chronic stress and inflammation could be two major factors for several of my autoimmune diseases, including my heart condition and eczema.

Some notable examples of my symptoms and healing trajectory include:

- Two front broken teeth, age 12
- Sinusitis, age 13
- Pharyngitis, age 14
- Broken tooth abscess, age 14
- Root canal therapy on two front teeth, age 19
- Immigrated to USA from India, age 23
- Root canal therapy redone in US, age 30
- High blood pressure, age 37
- Apicoectomy (a surgical procedure to correct a failed root canal), age 39
- Post-nasal drip and snoring, age 43
- Lack of proper sleep, age 43
- Fatigue and dark circles under eyes, age 45
- Recurring urinary tract infections, age 47
- Eczema, age 48
- Heart attack and subsequent angioplasty, age 55
- Congestive heart failure, age 59
- Gout, age 61
- Acute breathlessness and AICD implantation, age 64

- Ordered a MedicAlert® pendant for emergencies, age 64
- Extraction of two front teeth with dental bridge replacement, age 67
- Healthy heart (ejection fraction > 60), age 68
- No gout recurrence, age 69
- AICD intentionally disabled, age 71
- Eczema gone, age 72
- Sinus and pharynx clear, no snoring, age 72
- No dark circles under the eyes, healthier complexion, age 72

Today, at age 72, my heart's ejection fraction is normal, the AICD is disabled, eczema, sinusitis, and joint pain are gone, my eyes and complexion are clearer, and my medications have been reduced. I feel younger, energetic, livelier, and happier.

What I Learned

Around the time I had my heart attack, I began to research health and well-being. I wanted to understand what caused my descent into poor health and how I could live a healthier and more balanced life. With the encouragement of my doctor to change my lifestyle and reduce stress, I embarked on this path to discover what true well-being is and how to achieve it.

The body is a complex self-regulating organism intricately connected with the universe. Holistic balance is the key to our health and vitality; there is no *dis-ease* when all of the parts inside our body and outside work and dance in perfect balance and harmony.

Did chronic low-grade inflammation of the gum abscess aggravated by fast food and stress of modern life in America cause my chronic conditions? In retrospect, it seems very likely. Chronic nasopharyngitis owing to the abscess in the gums is an inflammatory process that can spread to the upper respiratory tract. It is caused by infections, including bacteria and fungi, and takes a long time to heal. In addition, heart disease owing to the inflammation of the gums has relevance in current medical research.

Information about inflammation and its relationship to weakened immune systems started to gain prominence in medical research at the turn of this century. I came to know about candida (yeast) overgrowth in 2000, and later in 2014 about the imbalance of our gut microbiome. Microbiome is the diverse trillions of bacteria, fungi, and viruses inhabiting our body and keeping us healthy when they are in balance. I learned that when our microbiome is out of balance it can cause various chronic diseases. Through my research, I was amazed to find that the rishis of India already had the intuitive knowledge of the microbiome in Ayurvedic medicine for more than five thousand years. Scientists in Western cultures rediscovered it only recently in 2007.

The foundation of Ayurveda is purity of body and mind (*saucha*). Inflammation in the body can be caused by the loss of the ecological diversity and balance of the microbiome. Discoveries related to the microbiome (post 2007) further confirm the Ayurvedic wisdom and candida overgrowth paradigm. According to the latest pundits and scientists of microbiota, "Richness of microbiota is key to health." (See Resources)

Researchers are amazed to find that microbiomes are unique to each individual and are dynamically affected by our lifestyle (food, diet, elimination, exercise, environment, thinking, mood, etc.), and yet any imbalance can cause various chronic diseases. A three-way interaction between genome, diet/lifestyle and the existing microbiota continuously shapes our health. Microbial diversity as well as ecologically balanced microbial community provides a smooth functioning, non-inflammatory organism, whereas less diversity or ecological imbalance can create chronic inflammatory conditions. These imbalances can be caused by drugs, sedentary lifestyle, inadequate nutrition, stress, and environmental factors. Antibiotics and immunosuppressants are also contributing factors that harm the microbiome. Physical as well as mental diseases are the consequences of these unstable environments.

Ayurveda prescribes a daily routine, *dinacharya*, for detoxification and cleansing of the body organs where our trillions of microbiome reside, for example, in the gut, oral and nasal cavities, eyes, and skin. The Ayurvedic system believes that problems with the digestive tract and the upper respiratory tract are the most common causes of the majority of diseases. Hence, Ayurveda places heavy emphasis on cleaning these tracts on a daily basis where our microbiomes primarily reside.

Now it is being discovered that microbiome imbalance in the gut can cause leaky gut or even leaky brain and a host of autoimmune disorders that were unknown fifty years ago. Heart disease, cancer, and diabetes are also being labeled as autoimmune diseases where the body becomes the raging battlefield to fight inflammation. Microbial imbalance creates inflammation throughout the body and causes the so-called "-itis" diseases. This suffix is used to create medical terms from Greek or Latin, for example, arthritis means inflammation of the joints.

According to Scripps Health (see Resources), the top ten health concerns of Baby Boomers are:

1. Type 2 diabetes
2. Heart disease (atherosclerosis)
3. Cancer
4. Depression
5. Eye problems
6. Alzheimer's disease
7. Arthritic joint replacement
8. Osteoporosis
9. Flu/pneumonia
10. Stress

Interestingly, all of the above noted conditions are caused by or can cause inflammation that is usually exacerbated by poor lifestyle. Chronic stress in itself can be a major cause of inflammation.

In the Ayurvedic tradition, the most important component of health is what we eat—food is a medicine. A balanced diet is personalized for each individual based on their unique characteristics called *doshas*. There are three kinds of *doshas*: *vata*, *pitta*, and *kapha*. The *doshas* are dynamic energies derived from the five elements—air, fire, water, earth, sky/space—that constitute our individual body and mind, and constantly change based on our inner and outer conditions. A person with distinctly *vata* constitution will have qualities of space and air, *pitta* reflects elements of fire and water, and *kapha* reflects elements of water and earth. Balance of *doshas* according to each individual's constitution of body and mind is the key to health and vitality in Ayurveda.

After consultation and examination by an Ayurvedic physician, you can fine-tune your diet to meet their recommendations. In this book, you will find ideas on how to achieve this goal that are generally applicable and can be considered as the common denominator across a broad cross-section of people. Of course, it is always best to consult with and follow your specific physician's recommendations.

Our ancestors knew that a balanced meal contains six tastes:

1. Sweet
2. Salty
3. Sour
4. Pungent
5. Bitter
6. Astringent

These tastes keep our bacteria (microbiome) healthy. In other words, a balanced meal keeps our *doshas—vata, kapha* and *pitta*—in check, which makes our immune system strong. Thus, our healthy bacteria are able to ward off chronic diseases. Spices and fermented food, also known as probiotics, provide astringent with salty, sour, and bitter taste, much needed for a healthy diet.

With all this knowledge, I took a dual-pronged naturopathic and integrative medicinal approach to heal my body. It took years, almost two decades, to turn my sinking ship toward healthy waters. In the summer of 2011, I moved to be near a spiritual community in a rural area to simplify my life and meditate more. This change in my lifestyle has been key to my healing. Apart from my integrative cardiologist of the past sixteen years, my health team includes a Tibetan Ayurvedic naturopath, an acupuncturist, a geriatric primary care physician, and my dentist. Today, my heart is healthy with an excellent ejection fraction above 60%, and the AICD was disabled more than a year ago. I take three generic prescription drugs and three supplements. I lead a normal healthy life. I am immensely grateful to my cardiologist for saving my life. Now, I am expanding my horizon to live a productive life for another twenty to thirty years—God willing!

What We Need

Ancient Ayurvedic wisdom has given us a clear prescription for a healthy and long life. So, what are those ingredients for good health and longevity?

- Daily personal hygiene routine
- Moderate and balanced diet with fresh and nutritious food
- Regular exercise
- Good sleep
- Open air
- Sunbathing
- Meditation
- Intermittent fasting
- Moderation in everything

"Continence, temperance and little care."

~Swami Sivananda

I believe that by modifying lifestyle, 85-90% of chronic conditions could be cured or averted. The good news is that these healthy habits are inexpensive. However, they take time and willpower to follow them.

The payoffs I have experienced have been tremendous. Everyone can benefit from this ancient wisdom. It is now my pleasure to share with you these Ayurvedic practices, tips, and insights that were essential on my healing journey with the wish that they will aid you toward full health and increased vitality. The effort is worth it because you will get your life back. This book is my humble effort toward this vision.

May you BE healthy!

How to Use This Book

Consider this book an owner's manual full of tips for taking good care of ourselves. Our bodies and minds are infinitely more complicated than any automobile we own. And yet, we may not be paying the needed attention to keep our food, water, and air filters clean, and to feed ourselves with the right octane fuel for maximum mileage.

This book is also designed to motivate and inspire you to self-reflect and critically think about your health habits and overall well-being, as well as gift you with the knowledge to start making lasting changes in your lifestyle and overall health.

Beyond the contents of this book, I encourage you to engage with other health experts and secondary sources, and when you are fortified with knowledge, commit this wisdom into actions that are right for you. Internet resources like Google or YouTube are also convenient and powerful for this purpose. Most importantly, always keep your health support team by your side.

This book is organized into four parts:

PART I: Everyday Health Practices
PART II: Homemade Healing Products
PART III: Healthy Cooking Guidelines and Recipes
PART IV: Living Your Healthiest Life

PART I Everyday Health Practices is the core of this book. Each chapter details how to instill sound cleansing, food, exercise, and meditation practices to help you build a supportive health team.

PART II describes simple and inexpensive ways for making natural homemade healing products for personal use.

PART III includes recipes and guidelines for cooking and eating healthy meals.

PART IV provides additional resources and references including a checklist of important healthy habits.

As you read this knowledge and assimilate ideas into practice, I recommend following these guidelines to help you gain the maximum benefit:

1. Read, critically think, and take time to understand the content.
2. Commit yourself to a healthy lifestyle.
3. Understand the benefits and challenges of each recommended habit or procedure.
4. Research and practice the new habit or procedure.
5. Start slowly, change only a few habits at a time.
6. Monitor your progress with introspection or keep a diary.
7. Ask questions.
8. Plan to fail sometimes. It is normal. When you do, simply pick yourself up again like a toddler does while learning to walk.
9. Celebrate your milestones, even the small ones, by rewarding yourself when you establish a good habit.
10. Always be grateful. Create a supportive environment.
11. Learn to experiment.
12. Know that all these good habits are investments for a healthy life.

A checklist of important habits is shown in PART IV to implement in your daily life. How do we successfully incorporate a new good habit? One creative approach would be to attach a new daily or weekly activity to an established ritual to increase the chance of its completion. Example: I shall eat my snack, one serving of seasonally fresh fruit in the morning after breakfast or after my afternoon nap. Visualize a reward or outcome—a lighter you!—or treat yourself to a cup of tea or coffee. Take only a few new habits at a time using a Swiss cheese approach whereby you make small holes into a larger chunk to gradually make a significant difference.

Daily Log for Monitoring a New Habit

Calendar Days	Habit #1 Detox	Habit #2 Food	Habit #3 Exercise	Habit #4 Meditation
Jan 1st	Yes or No			
Jan 2nd				
.....				

Create a daily log to monitor your performance in a simple Yes (Y) or No (N) fashion. Be non-judgmental.

When you have missed it, try again. In silence, visualize the new habits in action and contemplate upon the physical benefits. Absorb it into your subconscious mind. The good news is that after practicing a new habit for three weeks or more, it will become easier and natural. As you are able to gradually purify your body and your mind through healthy living, you'll find yourself happier and more energetic.

This book is not about winning or being perfect. It is about seeking your own balance. This book supports you in being constantly proactive in living a healthy lifestyle. You don't need to be perfect in each habit that you undertake. The improvements will come gradually and naturally. Enjoy the process and the well-being you are creating for yourself. You will be amazed with the life-changing results.

PART I

Everyday Health Practices

"He who indulges daily in healthy food and activities, who discriminates the good and bad of everything and then acts wisely, who is not attached [too much] to the objects of the senses, who develops the habit of charity, of considering all as equal [requiring kindness], of truthfulness, of pardoning, and keeping company of good persons only, becomes free from all diseases."

~Astanga Hrdayam

Genes play a role in keeping us healthy, but lifestyle is more important for good health. In fact, nurture is more important than nature, though according to the new research called "epigenetics," they are connected.

Our lifestyle accounts for 90% of health, our DNA, only 10%. This is great news. It is highly empowering. It is also consistent with age-old wisdom, as well as new age thinking. We are in control of our body and mind. We are what we eat. We are what we think.

Our body is our vehicle that takes us around to accomplish our goals in life. This vehicle needs to perform reliably. Like caring for an automobile, as its owner we must perform the required periodic maintenance, feed it the right fuel, wash and wax often, and drive responsibly on the road of life.

In this section, I explain age-old Ayurvedic techniques to keep the body clean internally and externally by detoxifying and washing, by moving, stretching and exercising, and eating mostly fresh plant-based food.

The root words for "health" and "healing" are "whole," "hale" and "holy." Ayurveda is a holistic approach to health and vitality. Ayurveda always strives for the balance in body and mind as the foundation for optimum health. Modern medicine has started to realize this fact.

"The key to good health may lie in finding the right balance between the body's intricate pro-inflammatory and anti-inflammatory forces."

~William Meggs, MD,
Author, *Inflammation Cure*

Chapter 1

Daily and Natural Detoxification

In Ayurveda, the prescription for a healthy life consists of:

1. *Saucha,* meaning purity of body and mind.
2. *Dinacharya, meaning* daily routine for purification (detoxification) of body and mind.
3. *Yoga*, meaning union of body, mind, and spirit, and signifiying a state of higher consciousness of peace, equanimity, and bliss.

These cleansing practices are beneficial for alleviating and preventing all chronic diseases of the body and mind. Each practice is designed to daily cleanse the internal or external organs where microbiome reside, for example, the gastrointestinal tract, mouth, nose, eyes, and skin. The ecological balance of the diverse microbial community is the key to our strong immune system. Ayurveda called it the balance of *doshas*: *vata* (air), *pitta* (fire), and *kapha* (earth) qualities.

Eight Morning Cleaning Rituals

Dinacharya consists of eight morning rituals. They are recommended to clean your body temple before offering it food or breakfast. Breakfast is actually the breaking of the 12-16 hours of fasting from the previous night's supper. A prescribed set of daily cleaning is highly recommended before our first meal of the day.

The rituals are:

1. Early to rise and shine.
2. Regular bowel movement.
3. Head-to-toe self-massage.
4. Oil pulling.
5. Washing eyes, ears, and mouth.
6. Nasal irrigation, and ear and nose lubrication.
7. Teeth brushing, tongue scraping, and flossing.
8. Shaving, showering, and towel scrubbing/drying.

The above-noted daily detoxification activities are known as Ayurvedic *saucha* practices.

Although Ayurveda recommends all these practices to be performed early in the morning after waking up, you can divide some of these practices throughout your day to suit your lifestyle. The most effective times to complete these practices are early morning and before going to sleep. We need to assess our current cleansing habits and when we do them. Select how you wish to incorporate these new cleansing practices into your daily cleansing routine.

As you adopt these habits, notice how your health changes. Some of these rituals will cure both recurrent and chronic health issues over time. Your hair and skin may become softer. Your nails may start to get their luster back, and you may start to enjoy calmness and even enjoy mealtimes more.

Helpful Tools

To effectively perform these practices, you will need to acquire some tools for your detoxifying morning routine. All of these tools are common, inexpensive, and easy to find. You will most likely already have some, but others may be new to you.

- Comb
- Cup or glass

- Dental floss
- Distilled water
- Electric pot or mug warmer
- Eye dropper
- Eye wash cup
- Herbal powder (neem, psyllium, and triphala)
- Herbal soap
- Massage oils (coconut or sesame)
- Neti pot
- Sea salt
- Soft skin brush
- Teaspoons (2)
- Tongue scraper
- Toothbrush
- Toothpowder (herbal) or natural toothpaste

Morning Cleaning Ritual #1
Early to Rise and Shine

Frequency: Daily

Waking before the sun rises is the ancient wisdom of our ancestors. We are a vital part of nature and our health is interdependent on our daily circadian rhythm connected to the sun and the moon. By rising before the sun and by completing our daily cleaning rituals, we are now ready to undertake other activities and work efficiently during the day. Try to gradually adjust yourself to rising early if your work schedule permits.

How to practice:

1. As you wake, relax in your bed for a few minutes.
2. Your mind is still very calm from sleep. Observe your quiet mind.
3. Stretch from head to toe, about 2-3 times.

4. When you feel ready, slowly rise from your bed.
5. While standing, feel your belly with both hands breathing up and down. Do this for a minute.
6. Rub your hands briskly and then touch your face and eyes with your warm palms.
7. Soak yourself with the rising sun with a short five-minute meditation facing the sun or preferably to the east, where possible. This directly sets the circadian clock and regulates your rhythm for the day ahead.

Morning Cleaning Ritual #2
Regular Bowel Movement

Frequency: Daily

Developing a habit of fully evacuating your bowel immediately after waking up in the morning is a vital component to overall well-being and an age-old essential Ayurvedic daily purification (*saucha dinacharya*) practice. By doing this regularly, you are ridding your body of waste and toxins.

Most of us have forgotten in the daily humdrum of modern life about the disciplined first training we received from our mothers—being toilet-trained to regularly evacuate our bowel.

It is vital to keep your gut clean, home to 70% of your microbiome. Lack of microbial imbalance as well as diversity in our gut is the major cause of various inflammations that can create chronic disease of body and mind. A clean gut is the essential requirement for health and vitality according to Ayurveda.

How to practice:

1. Upon waking, drink a glass of warm water with lemon.
2. Bend to touch your knees to facilitate bowel movement.
3. The urge to eliminate waste and urine should be obeyed promptly and not delayed. As needed, you may take a mild Ayurvedic laxative to assist this natural daily movement. Triphala capsules or psyllium

husk dissolved in warm water are the most gentle and effective. They are best taken the night before at bedtime to aid the bowel movement for the following morning.

4. Notice and record the frequency, regularity, color, shape, and density of your bowel movements. Record also the frequency and color of urine, especially a few days before your appointment with your holistic doctor. This is important because your naturopath can use this information to assess the health of your gut, kidneys, and liver.

Morning Cleaning Ritual #3
Head-to-Toe Self-Massage

Frequency: Daily

Give yourself a head-to-toe massage every day preferably with oil, though your dry palms will suffice. If daily practice is not possible, do this at least once a week. Ayurvedic massage from a therapist can be done if needed for painful joints, but it is expensive and time-consuming. Regular self-massage is a good habit for detoxification, prevention of disease, aiding with joint pains, and for maintaining soft and glowing skin.

This is the age-old Ayurvedic skin purification practice. Skin is the largest organ in our body. Fifteen percent of your microbiome lives on your skin. Skin and joints become hydrated, glowing, and free of inflammation when massaged. Dry skin brushing or oil massage decreases cellulite and cleans the lymphatic system.

Oil is deeply revered in Ayurveda. Coconut oil, sesame oil, almond oil, and ghee can be used. Shower with lukewarm water after the oil massage. Otherwise, you may use a dry brush or a silk cloth to brush skin from head to toe, including nose, ears, face, hair, and nails.

How to practice:

1. Put 1-2 teaspoons of oil on your palms. Use sesame oil in the winter and coconut oil in the summer.
2. Rub the oil slowly under your feet, and across your toes, then over your fingers and nails.

3. Massage your entire body by briskly rubbing both your palms over your skin for at least five minutes.
4. With your index finger, rub oil onto both your navel and ear openings with a circular motion.
5. Once you have completed your self-massage, take a warm shower and rinse off the oil.

Morning Cleaning Ritual #4
Oil Pulling

Frequency: Daily

Almost 15% of your microbiome lives in your oral cavity. Therefore, it is imperative to keep this area clean. The results from oil pulling include cleaner, brighter, and shinier teeth as well as cleaner, healthier gums and joints. It is reported that regular oil pulling can reduce cavities and also decrease gum inflammation. It strengthens teeth and can even improve your sense of taste and strengthen your voice.

How to practice:

1. Place a tablespoon of oil in your mouth. Use sesame oil in the winter and coconut oil in the summer.
2. Swish the oil around in your mouth for 5-7 minutes, moving it around the oral cavity. The oil will become thick. Do not swallow.
3. When the time is up, spit the oil out in the sink. Spit coconut oil into a separate container to avoid clogging the sink.
4. Rinse out your mouth with warm water to eliminate any residue from the oil.
5. Brush your teeth afterwards.

Note: If you do not feel comfortable swishing oil around your mouth, you can do the same thing by swishing warm water with acceptable results, which is called water pulling.

Tip: You may find oil pulling while sitting on the toilet a good use of your time.

Morning Cleaning Ritual #5
Washing Your Eyes, Ears, and Mouth (Oral Microbiome)

Frequency: Daily

The next four cleansing steps are related to cleansing your oral microbiome where trillions of bacteria live and work for you. It is important to consult your primary care physician or ENT (Ear, Nose, Throat) specialist about cleansing the nose and ears as recommended here.

How to practice:

1. Wash or splash your face with cold water only. You can use an eye cup to wash each eye with water a couple of times. Develop the habit of blinking your eyes often.
2. Wash both the nasal and oral cavity by blowing away any accumulated mucus.
3. Swish some clean water in your mouth, gargle and throw it out forcefully without swallowing it
4. Briskly massage your ear openings in a rotating motion with your index finger to clear any ear wax debris.
5. Use a cotton hand towel to pat your face dry.

Morning Cleaning Ritual #6
Nasal Irrigation (Neti)

Frequency: Daily

Nasal irrigation is an easy and safe way to gradually cleanse your sinuses and heal them from inflammation. In Ayurveda, this cleansing process is called neti, a Sanskrit word.

Neti clears the nasal passages, improves breathing, and may help to reduce and even prevent snoring, sleep apnea, and dry eyes. Nasal irrigation was approved by the American Medical Association in 2004, though like the rest of these eight morning rituals, it is an ancient Ayurvedic practice (5,000 BC). Local pharmacy shops sell disposable nasal bottles and syringes for this purpose. The neti pot is my favorite because it is reliable, simple, inexpensive, and reusable. A neti pot looks like a small teapot with an upward pointing spout.

How to use the neti pot:

1. Pour warm water into the neti pot (not too hot or cold) until almost full. Distilled water is preferable. Add a pinch of sea salt and swirl to dissolve before use.
2. Facing the sink, tilt your head sideways and downward so your head is low enough for water to flow from the pot slowly into the top facing nostril. The water will flow out of the lower nostril into the sink.
3. Repeat several times.
4. Turn your head the other way and repeat this nasal cleansing process for the other nostril.
5. Use a small amount of remaining saline water to gargle and expel any remaining mucous.

After completing the nasal irrigation process, bend forward and touch your toes a couple of times to drain the water from the nostrils.

Ear and Nose Lubrication (*Nasya*)

Frequency: Daily

Ear and nose openings can be lubricated after cleaning. Consult your primary care physician or ENT specialist about the lubrication of nose and ears with oil as recommended here.

How to practice:

1. Place sesame oil on your index finger and then into each nostril. Apply similarly to the ear openings. Another method is to put 2-4 drops of almond oil, ghee, or sesame oil in each nostril and inhale with a snort to lubricate the nasal passages.
2. Once a week, say Sunday, tilt your head to the side and add 2-4 drops of oil into each ear opening to allow the oil to enter the ear passage and lubricate the eardrum.

Morning Cleaning Ritual #7
Teeth Brushing, Tongue Scraping, and Flossing

Frequency: Daily

Keep your tongue clean and your teeth white and plaque-free by regularly brushing your teeth and flossing followed by a tongue scraping. These daily activities improve your oral microbiome and keep your teeth and gums healthy.

How to practice:

1. Using an Ayurvedic tooth powder (see recipe in PART II), place a quarter teaspoon in your left palm, add half a teaspoon of sesame oil, and rub into a paste with your right index finger.
2. Use your finger to apply this paste to your teeth and along the inner and outer side of your lower and upper gums.
3. Massage the paste along the gums and into the crevices and ridges inside your mouth.
4. Brush your teeth and gums with a toothbrush and thoroughly rinse your mouth.
5. Perform these steps every morning and night before bed.
6. You can finish brushing with your favorite flavored toothpaste if you like. Next, use a u-shaped tongue scraper made of stainless steel or copper to gently scrape your tongue in a forward and backward motion. This will remove the deposits in the upper surface of the tongue.
7. Wash your tongue scraper for reuse the next morning.
8. Floss at least once in the morning, preferably also at night.

Tip: In Ayurveda, a twig from a neem tree is used to make a disposable toothbrush by chewing the end and brushing with it. After brushing, the twig is split in half and used as a tongue scraper before disposing. It is a remarkable biodegradable toothbrush and tongue scraper all in one.

Morning Cleaning Ritual #8
Shaving, Showering, and Towel Scrubbing/Drying

Frequency: Daily

A shower washes off toxins from the skin and is invigorating. Also, taking a shower is necessary after you have given yourself a head-to-toe massage with oil.

How to practice:

1. Shower with warm water, slightly above body temperature, from the collar bones down. Clean the perineum, anus, and urinary area with natural soap only. It is not advisable to use soap on the whole body every day because soap makes the skin dry.
2. Many people prefer to shave in the shower or you can shave before entering the shower.
3. Use water at a cooler temperature, close to body temperature, for washing your hair and scalp. Never use very hot water on the head or other parts of your body because hot water can scald your skin and make it dry. The same is true for the scalp and hair.
4. At the end of your shower, turn the water to cold for about 30-60 seconds. This will invigorate your lymph nodes and all your body cells, as well as build resilience in handling adverse situations by helping you to keep calm.
5. After your shower, use a rough and thin cotton towel to vigorously scrub as well as dry your whole body.

Frame Your Day

Just a couple of minutes setting your intention for the day can have a powerful impact on both the subconscious and conscious mind. You will become more effective and aware as a result of this simple habit.

You can begin in your shower. Visualize and frame your day with an optimistic curiosity for the way it will unfold. One way to do this would be to rehearse the events as if you are alert in a lucid dreaming state. Be aware of your state of consciousness. Are you calm? Or are you restless? Something in between? Notice this and see if you can reframe your thoughts and feelings.

After you complete your daily morning cleaning routine, look at yourself in the mirror. Check to see that your face, nasal cavities and ears have no remaining unwanted particles. Inspect your whole face—eyes, eyelids, lips, tongue, teeth. If you have done a good job with cleansing, your face will exude balance and inner health. Congratulations!

Now, it is important to stretch a little to get movement and energy flowing in your body. This is accomplished with two breathing exercises: *Anulom Vilom* and *Kapalbhati*. These yoga asanas incorporate breathing with a short meditation. An explanation of these breathing exercises can be found in the section on yoga asanas in Chapter 4.

Now it is time to break your fast. Ideally, do so with sprouted mung beans, as they are good prebiotics, vital for a healthy gut. Mix them with a tablespoon of fermented vegetables. Choose from a variety, like sauerkraut or kimchi. Drink a cup of homemade kefir (a probiotic) topped with one teaspoon freshly ground flaxseed, chia seed, and unshelled pumpkin seed. Ground shell-on pumpkin seeds add more fiber. All of these are gluten-free and contain vital nutrients, specifically short chain fatty acids, omega-3s, soluble and insoluble fiber, and antioxidants. I never leave home without this breakfast combo.

With your gut flora fortified, you can have your regular breakfast—one egg a day is okay—with coffee or tea. An ideal lunch consists of one-third raw fresh salad, one-third cooked vegetables, and one-third entree of your choice, ideally a plant-based selection. Breakfast and lunch should be the main meals of your day. Keep supper light, preferably freshly made soup or a healthy comfort food. Comfort foods are easy to digest, and liquid or smooth in texture, for example, soup or khichdi. Eat your last meal before 7 p.m. For exercise, walk 3-4 miles each day and do a short yoga or stretch session in the evening followed by meditation before a good night sleep.

Here is an example of an ideal framework that incorporates all of the morning rituals and routine activities for a normal day. Of course, you can modify this to fit your unique needs.

Sample Ideal Daily Framework

Time	Activities	Remarks
5:00 a.m.	Wake-up	Stay in bed quietly for 5 minutes; stretch head to toe before leaving the bed.
5:00 a.m.	Drink a glass of warm water	Touch toes and walk a few steps before doing the daily cleansing routine for 45-60 minutes.
5:00-6:15 a.m.	*Dinacharya*	Toilet evacuation, head-to-toe self-massage, oil pulling, eye wash, neti, *nasya*, teeth brushing, tongue cleaning, flossing, shaving, and shower.
6:15-7:15 a.m.	Yoga asana and meditation	Chew a few neem leaves. Drink a glass of warm water with lemon before prayers.
7:15-7:45 a.m.	Break Fast	Half apple, sprouted mung beans with fermented vegetables, kefir with fresh flaxseed, chia seed, ground pumpkin seeds, and walnuts, one poached egg, and tea.
8:00-noon	Work	Job tasks, reading, writing, news, emails, fruit; few nuts and coffee as a snack.
Noon-12:30 p.m.	Personal meditation	Sunbathing while meditating.
12:30-1:00 p.m.	Lunch	Mostly plant based.
1:00-5:00 p.m.	Work	Reading, writing, computer, phone calls. Include a snack consisting of fruit or whole grains and tea.

Continued...

Time	Activities	Remarks
5:00-6:00 p.m.	Movement	Yoga, walking, swimming, or some other form of movement/exercise.
6:00-6:30 p.m.	Personal meditation	Breathing exercise plus meditation.
6:30-7:00 p.m.	Supper	Enjoy soup or light comfort food.
7:00-9:30 p.m.	Renew and connect	Read, reflect, journal, listen to music, and write thank you notes.

Chapter 2

Food is Medicine

"Let food be thy medicine, and medicine be thy food."

~Hippocrates

As Hippocrates so famously said, food is medicine. A well-balanced diet must supply the various constituents of food in adequate quantity and it must yield proper caloric content. You do not have to spend lots of money to get a well-balanced diet, but you must know how to prepare one. You need to gain knowledge about wholesome food. A lot of this wisdom is common sense that has been available to our ancestors in all cultures. Therefore, you want to make sure that your food is made with fresh and pure ingredients and is customized to your needs. You want to eat "slow food" not "fast food." Cooking at home can be fun and less expensive. A simple, wholesome, well-balanced meal is much better than rich restaurant food that is not well-balanced where you also do not know how the food was prepared or the freshness of the ingredients. Cooking is an art. Planning a meal, cooking, and eating together can be wholesome fun.

After cleaning and detoxifying your body through daily practice, you will want to eat healthy food to keep your microbiome nourished.

What are the Basics of a Healthy Diet?

The desire for a healthy diet is universal and is based on the following simple principles:

- Eat fresh, local, and a variety of primarily plant-based foods that are nutrient-dense and contain ample phytonutrients and fiber.
- Aim for 6 servings a day of fruits and vegetables (raw and cooked).
- Eat around 30 or more varieties of fruits, veggies, nuts, and legumes each week to build a diverse gut microbiome.
- Include a variety of whole grains and legumes for protein and complex carbohydrates.
- Incorporate good fats from oil, ghee, nuts, and seeds.
- Eat a minimum of animal protein; one egg per day is fine.
- Avoid sugar and processed food.

How Much is One Serving?

Simply put, one serving is the same size of your closed fist. This easy-to-use measurement naturally takes into account your age, build, genetic makeup, and even gender.

For cooked vegetables and fruits, you only need half the amount to make a serving. Technically, a one-cup measure equals one serving as does one-half cup cooked vegetables or fruit. For example, one apple or orange is one serving. One cup of leafy green spinach or one half cup of cooked spinach equals one serving.

The Importance of Prebiotic and Probiotic Foods

What are prebiotics and probiotics? Prebiotics are food for our bacteria while probiotics are about populating our gastrointestinal tract with good bacteria.

Fibrous fruits and cruciferous vegetables are good prebiotic foods. They keep the tract clean by helping to maintain regular bowel movements. More fiber in your diet also reduces cholesterol, triglycerides, blood glucose, and improves your overall microbiome.

Some examples of healthy prebiotic foods include:

- Apples
- Artichokes
- Beets
- Berries
- Broccoli
- Brussels sprouts
- Cauliflower
- Jicama
- Leafy greens
- Lentils
- Onions
- Radishes
- Sprouted beans
- Sweet potatoes

Be sure to include at least two of these prebiotic foods with each meal. When eating out, choose a salad bar that provides a lot of these healthy foods.

Cultured or fermented foods are good sources of probiotics since they populate the intestinal tract with beneficial bacteria. Antibiotics ingested through prescription drugs, meat, and eggs, devastate and deplete the bacterial colonies in our gut. Probiotics replenish them.

Healthy probiotic foods include:

- Buttermilk
- Cottage cheese
- Fermented veggies (sauerkraut, kimchi)
- Ghee (clarified butter)
- Kefir (Bulgarian sour milk)

- Indian cottage cheese (chenna)
- Pickles
- Yogurt

Make sure to include at least one probiotic rich food with each meal. When eating out include cottage cheese or yogurt.

Why Eat Fermented Foods?

The short answer is for good health. Homemade probiotics and fermented veggies are essential foods to replenish and build the diversity of our gut microbiome. Our ancestors knew about this. Every culture has devoted time to prepare fermented foods, be it bread, yogurt, cheese, kefir, injera, dosa, kimchi, sauerkraut, or pickles. Unfortunately, in the quick-paced modern world of fast foods, slow fermented food has been greatly diminished and our ancestor's wisdom has been set aside.

Eat a variety of fermented food throughout the week. Fermentation or culturing of food takes time. Bacteria multiply in a favorable environment. These bacteria or microbes are part of trillions of cells inhabited in our bodies to keep us healthy. When we lack these vital microbes, we become imbalanced and more susceptible to chronic diseases including: allergies, Alzheimer's, asthma, cancer, heart disease, and obesity. This is the most stunning discovery in medicine in the last decade. Our microbiome is much more important than our genes in keeping us healthy.

It is not surprising that our ancestors knew this basic truth. Gut health is the key for maintaining overall well-being. In addition, the gut, brain, and all other organs are directly connected to our microbiome. Truly, we are what we eat.

We are now finding out that fermented foods, including milk products such as cheese have been an important part in this microbiome balancing puzzle for people all around the world. The reward in eating these types of foods has been increased health and vitality for our ancestors. We need to recover this ancient wisdom and move away from the modern world of fast food. The processed food experiment of the last seventy years has degenerated our health and vitality.

Homemade Probiotics

Probiotics are live foods with prana or chi (life force energy). They keep our gut microbiome diverse, which makes our immunity strong.

Freshly made yogurt or kefir are more powerful in bacteria strength compared to the ones bought in a store. These can be blended with different milks (vegan or dairy). Blended milk kefirs are not easily available in grocery stores, but they are both inexpensive and easy to make at home. Of course, you can buy fermented vegetables to complement these, for example, kimchi, sauerkraut, wasabi, and pickles. However, if you can, it is often best to make your own.

Here are a few suggestions to improve your diet regimen:

1. Make fresh yogurt or kefir daily and eat one serving with your breakfast. This is a powerful probiotic.
2. Make your own mung bean and chana sprouts for a powerful breakfast prebiotic.

Here is a sample menu for prebiotic and probiotic foods.

Breakfast

- Homemade kefir (organic cow's or goat milk, non-dairy, or even water kefir).
- Sprouted mung beans with fermented vegetables and omega-3s in the form of seeds and nuts.
- One egg, boiled or poached.

Snacks

- Fruits.
- Whole grain crackers with cottage cheese.
- Coffee/tea (optional).

Lunch

- Mix sprouted mung beans and a few pieces of fermented vegetables or a pickle with salad greens.
- Use kefir as salad dressing. Alternatively, drink a cup of kefir with digestive herbs, for example, roasted and powdered cumin, fennel, ajwain (carom), and Himalayan salt.

Alkaline and Low-Glycemic (Low Sugar) Foods

Alkaline foods keep your gastrointestinal tract clean. Low-glycemic index foods have fewer simple carbohydrates and therefore do not overload your pancreas with insulin production. As a general rule, plant-based foods are alkaline whereas animal products, soda, alcohol, tea, and coffee are acidic.

Alkaline and low-glycemic index foods are non-inflammatory, protect your gut lining, help keep it clean, and nourish your overall body.

Examples of healthy low-glycemic low-sugar foods:

- Apples
- Citrus fruits
- Guavas
- Legumes
- Lemons
- Nuts
- Whole grains* (except refined rice)
- Vegetables (except potatoes)

*Indian dal, split pea, lima bean, Bengal gram (white chickpea), whole mung bean, quinoa, Besan (chana dal flour from split brown chickpea), or basmati rice.

Sugar and processed foods are best avoided because they are acidic and have very high glycemic index (GI) values. Though meat and fish have low GI values, eating fewer animal products is desirable because they are acidic in nature, contain toxins, and are naturally high in cholesterol. You can reward yourself once a while with a candy, cookie, or a dessert only after you have eaten a good low GI meal as a foundation, but never on an empty stomach.

Where Do I Find Information on Food and its Gi Value?

There are many excellent references. I recommend the Glycemic Index website (www.glycemicindex.com). You can search for a food and find its GI value.

Foods with high GI values raise blood glucose levels more than those with low or medium values. They are useful for dietary variety and for replenishing muscle fuel stores after strenuous exercise. For people with diabetes who have low blood glucose levels—hypoglycemia—high GI foods can quickly bring blood glucose levels back to normal. Foods with low GI values are useful to include in each meal to lower the overall GI of the diet. Following a low GI diet is associated with better long-term health.

Where Do I Find Information on Alkaline Food and its pH Value?

You can go to the pH Miracle website (www.phmiracle.com) and browse through foods that range from very alkaline to very acidic to form a general idea of foods to eat whether you cook at home or eat out.

What are Phytonutrients and How Do You Get Them?

Phytonutrients are special plant nutrients that help prevent disease and keep your body working properly.

Phytonutrients are found in plant foods: fruits, vegetables, beans, grains, including fresh and raw cruciferous vegetables. Seasonal fruits have the highest number of phytonutrients, and the levels decrease as the fruits decay. Optimize your intake of phytonutrients by eating a fresh variety of live plant foods.

Cruciferous Vegetables

Cruciferous vegetables are a family of vegetables with cross-shaped flowers, thus their name. They are high in vitamin C, soluble fiber, and contain multiple nutrients and phytochemicals.

Cruciferous vegetables include:

- Arugula
- Bok choy
- Broccoli
- Brussels sprouts
- Cabbage
- Cauliflower
- Greens (collard, mustard, turnip)
- Kale
- Kohlrabi
- Radishes
- Rutabaga
- Turnips
- Watercress

These foods are all rich in anticancer properties. They are best eaten raw or mildly cooked with their natural juices.

How Much Fiber Do I Need in My Diet?

Dietary fiber is a plant-based nutrient that passes through the intestinal tract relatively intact, acting as a cleanser as it passes through your system. Fiber can be soluble or insoluble, and both have benefits. Soluble fiber decreases blood sugar levels and insoluble fiber helps maintain the regularity of bowel movements. More is generally better. Depending on your specific health needs, consume at least 30 grams a day with one-third soluble. This amount promotes healthy bowel movements, reduces cholesterol, and maintains healthy blood sugar levels.

A serving of fruit or vegetables contain 2 grams of fiber on average, of which almost 50% is soluble. A serving of legumes contains 3 grams of fiber on average and is almost 50% soluble. Soluble fibers are also called prebiotics, which are necessary foods to maintain the health of your microbiome. Therefore, it is important to eat as many fruits, vegetables, and whole grains as possible. Keeping the skins on certain fruits and vegetables is another way to increase your fiber intake. Foods that are beneficial to eat with skins on are:

- Apples
- Baked or boiled potatoes and sweet potatoes
- Berries and cherries
- Carrots
- Eggplant
- Guavas
- Kumquats
- Loquats
- Nectarines
- Peaches
- Tomatoes

Tip: For an excellent and easy source of fiber, keep a mixture of flaxseeds, chia seeds, and pumpkin seeds in a jar. Freshly grind one tablespoon of this mixture and sprinkle it on your favorite dal, kefir drink, salad, or soup. You can also take psyllium husk and triphala powder as a fiber rich laxative to aid your bowel movements, if needed.

Chapter 3

Healthy Food Habits

In this chapter, you will find pointers and practical tips to eat healthy food at home or away from home. Here are fifty nifty ways to establish healthy food habits.

1. Foods boost mood. Eat only when hungry.
2. Every culture has perfected the art of eating over the ages. Learn from your ancestors.
3. Food is sacred. Pray before taking meals.
4. Eat real food. Eat 30 or more plant-based foods each week for a healthy microbiome.
5. Eat low-glycemic and alkaline foods. Eat a rainbow of colors. Eat leafy greens daily. Eat cruciferous vegetables often.
6. Eat fresh, eat local, eat whole, eat organic, eat a variety, eat seasonal, and rotate foods during the week.
7. Eat less meat. Eggs are okay for breakfast.
8. Eat salad (raw vegetables) with lunch.
9. Eat a serving of ripe fruit as an in between meal snack.
10. Use olive oil for salads, and ghee or butter for cooking; sesame oil, coconut oil or mustard oil for cooking if you are vegan—they contain good fat.

11. Use oil in cooking with discretion—it has high calories per gram. The Vedic recipes noted here use oil and spices in healthy combinations.
12. Eat a variety of prebiotic and probiotic foods and fermented vegetables.
13. Eat good fats high in omega-3s—olive oil with salad, ghee or sesame oil (vegan) for crackling garnish on soups.
14. Avoid processed foods like bottled drinks or products that include white flour or sugar. Shop on the periphery of a grocery store.
15. Eat slowly. Chew thoughtfully.
16. Store whole spices. Grind them in a coffee grinder before use.
17. Cook your meals at home as much as you can. Eat out selectively.
18. When eating out, order your food with the guidelines learned here: fresh, mostly plant-based foods, legumes for protein. Limit eggs, meat, and processed foods. Stay away from soda and drink water at room temperature. Tea and coffee are okay.
19. Learn to think about food in a creative way. Experiment with new recipes.
20. Make gradual changes. Start with breakfast. Eggs, bacon, donuts, white toast, or bagels can be switched to oatmeal, bran cereal, and fruit. If you can't spare minutes for a sit-down breakfast, grab high-fiber cereal bars instead of donuts or muffins. Next, try out salads, low-fat yogurt or low-fat cottage cheese, tuna or peanut butter sandwiches, and fruit for lunch. Snack on unsalted nuts, trail mix, fruit, raw vegetables, rye crisps, or graham crackers. Try eating a few handfuls of a crunchy fiber cereal.
21. Simplify cooking, rotate vegetables and whole grains for variety; garnish or season them with crackling spices and fresh herbs (preferably from your garden). Spices and herbs are anticarcinogenic, anti-inflammatory, and are a natural antidepressant. They are also soothing to your digestive system and add flavor.
22. Don't count calories strictly, but be prudent. Calories can vary depending on your physical work and your metabolism.

23. Shop for fresh food at farmers' markets and local co-ops. Look at websites and phone apps mentioned in the Resources section in the back of this book.
24. Know the freshness of your produce. The phytonutrients in fresh vegetables and fruits begin to decay within hours.
25. Eat breakfast like a king or queen. Eat lunch like a prince or princess. Eat a light supper like a pauper.
26. Wash and gargle after meals. Clean your hands often, especially before and after meals.
27. Rest a while after lunch. Walk a mile or so after supper.
28. Do not eat or drink after 7 p.m. Fast for12-16 hours daily, the time after supper until you break fast.
29. Fast intermittently when you can by skipping a meal or two in a row. Fast a day on orange juice once a week. People with diabetes or other ailments must seek a physician's advice before undertaking any fast or skipping meals.
30. Shop for yellow fresh vegetables in season because they are rare: pumpkin, yellow squash, and yellow bell pepper. Carrots, raw or boiled, are close substitutes and are easily available. Cabbage is greenish-yellow and can be eaten raw, cooked, or fermented.
31. Eat dessert only after the meal, preferably at lunch, because of its high glycemic value.
32. Drink water at room temperature between meals.
33. Minimize drinking water with meals. It weakens digestion and promotes allergies.
34. Avoid fruit juice; eat whole fruit instead.
35. Avoid cold drinks—no ice with tea or water.
36. Eat corn, soy, peanuts, eggs, cheese, fish, chicken, and meat in moderation.
37. Water is the best beverage, but coconut water at room temperature is also good if you crave a sweet drink.

38. Prepare a couple of glasses of herbal tea by boiling the water for a minute and cool it to room temperature to sip throughout the day.
39. Avoid soda, candy, sweets, artificial sweeteners, sweetened juice, and alcohol.
40. Eat fruit before or after meals as a snack, not with meals.
41. Eat a balanced diet: one-third salad, one-third vegetables, and one-third entree.
42. Never overeat; eating slowly fills you comfortably.
43. Avoid adding table salt to food.
44. Limit self-added sugar to no more than 5-6 teaspoons for 2-3 cups of tea or coffee.
45. Take unsulfured blackstrap molasses or honey as a substitute for sweeteners.
46. Talk to your grandparents about their cultural health habits.
47. After meals, do a quick 30-second water pulling (gargling) to clean the oral cavity. Take water in your mouth and move it around without swallowing for 30 seconds after meals. This age-old Vedic daily cleansing practice improves oral microbiome and prevents cavities.
48. Make cooking with kids and family members an interesting and creative project.
49. With the change of seasons, do a more rigorous detoxification or cleansing of your body including your digestive system and skin.
50. Skip a meal to give your digestive system a rest. Hunger with intermittent fasting is good for you.
    - Do a day fast on fruits and vegetables.
    - Do a day fast on freshly squeezed orange juice.
    - Do a day fast on water only.
    - Do a three-day fast on freshly squeezed orange juice.
    - Do a three-day fast on water, only under observation.

Creating a Healthy Pantry and Refrigerator

On the road to eating healthy, an important step is to clean out your pantry and refrigerator by discarding unhealthy foods and storing healthy ones in their place. This requires mindful attention and modification in purchasing and consumption of food items.

Cleaning Out Your Pantry and Refrigerator

Here are a few tips for making your pantry and refrigerator healthy and more vital spaces.

1. Take everything out of your refrigerator and pantry. Throw out all processed foods. Processed foods are unhealthy, usually high in salt, and high in simple carbohydrates/sugars (a high glycemic index).
2. Throw away condiments except vinegar and pickles. They age well.
3. Clean your fridge with soap and water, and repeat monthly. Avoid using harsh antimicrobial cleaners with triclosan.
4. Place only fresh food in fridge. It is best to use all your fresh food within the first few days. Fresh is best because vegetables and fruits lose their phytonutrients quickly. Phytonutrients fight disease and build your immunity.
5. Keep only whole grains in the pantry and a small amount of whole grain flour.
6. Keep only whole spices in the pantry. They remain fresh longer.
7. Keep fresh nuts, dry fruits, and seeds in small bottles at room temperature for use.
8. Keep your favorite fresh cookies, crackers, and dark chocolates as an infrequent snack.
9. Switch to a paper-free kitchen. Replace napkins with cloth towels.
10. Arrange for home delivery of organic fruits and vegetables. This will help you keep fresh produce in the house.

Tips for Acquiring Healthy Food

1. Grow your own herbs or buy fresh as needed.
2. Buy whole spices when you can and only grind the quantity needed for your recipe. You can buy them online in small amounts.
3. Buy a variety of whole grains, lentils, and legumes to last a couple of months. Store them in clear, airtight, space efficient glass containers.
4. Shop local when possible. Get to know your grocer. For best results, eat vegetables and fruits within three days of being plucked from the garden. The easiest way to do this is to grow your own and eat them fresh the day you pick them. When you shop for food, inquire about the freshness and location of the produce. Ask: how fresh, from where, and if it is organic.

Health-Giving Herbs and Spices

Spices are a healthy addition to your food if used moderately. Spices flavor food and are also beneficial as natural treatments against diseases owing to their antimicrobial properties. For example, turmeric (haldi), used in Indian curries for centuries, contains curcumin, now discovered to have many anti-inflammatory properties.

As compared to pharmaceutical drugs, spices are considered "nutraceuticals." Spices are made of the seeds, bark, stems, and roots of various plants and trees. They are dried for long-term food storage. Plant-based green herbs can be used for creating flavor, adding health benefits, and as a garnish.

Used in all cultures, spices preserve and flavor food. Dig into your grandma's cooking, gather recipes from traditional cookbooks, research on the Internet to enliven your culinary skills with their recipes and spices. Understand and observe how spices soothe your digestion, body, and mind daily. Fine tune the way you use spices with the changing seasons and place you live.

Crackling spices for tempering foods, especially dal and soups, is a creative as well as scientific art that you can experiment with for taste and healthiness. The same can be repeated for green herbs to garnish your food fresh from your garden.

Tip: Place herbs in an ice cube tray and fill it water and freeze it, storing it up to a few months. You can take one or two cubes out, thaw, and use to garnish your meal.

Nuts and Good Fat

Nuts are nutritious easy snacks. They are hearty, tasty, and rich in vitamin C, omega-3, vitamin D, selenium, B6, folate, zinc, and phytonutrients.

Nuts have oil, which is a good fat, but they are packed with calories. One tablespoon of nuts can have in excess of 100 calories. Therefore, eat nuts in moderation and eat a variety throughout the week.

Create a nut healthy snack by mixing almonds, Brazil nuts, cashews, peanuts, pistachios, and walnuts together. Take one handful daily of this nut mixture and add a few raisins or dried unsulfured figs, along with cranberries, blueberries, pomegranates, chia, flax, pumpkin seeds, and brewer's yeast.

Note: If you are allergic to nuts, eat the seeds and dried fruit and you will still have a nutritious snack.

Tips for Organizing Your Kitchen

Keeping food items visible where possible, labeling them, and using a bulletin board for reminders will help you stay organized and overall provide a more pleasant experience in your kitchen. Here are some tips that can help:

1. Organize and arrange your kitchen shelves to your cooking style. Make things visible in clear and airtight containers—rectangular are space efficient. Lazy Susan drawers and slide-out shelves are handy.
2. Keep a roll of masking tape and permanent markers, an 8" x 8" cork bulletin board, a dry erase white board, and scissors in your kitchen to make quick labels, post a recipe or jot down things to buy.

3. Place easily perishable salad items, fruits, and vegetables in your fridge at a visible location and use them fresh.
4. Buy a variety of legumes, lentils, and whole grains in sufficient quantity to last a couple of months. Store them in large, clear, air-tight, rectangular glass containers.
5. Soak legumes overnight before cooking to make them easier to digest. Simply put them in a bowl and cover them with water. Drain before use.

Special Tools for Your Kitchen

There are a few tools for your kitchen that will make cooking more efficient and fun. Invest in these inexpensive and easy-to-find simple gadgets.

1. Coffee grinder for spices (nuts and coffee).
2. Lazy Susan two-tier for spices.
3. Lazy Susan two-tier for nuts and seeds.
4. Garlic peeler: use a stainless spoon to remove skin from ginger and raw turmeric.
5. Onion chopper (for garlic, ginger, and raw turmeric).
6. Cast iron-skillet (3.5 inch) with lid.

Be sure to have pots and pans, good knives, and a food processor/ blender to help you prepare healthy meals. Consider investing in an Instant Pot (multi-use programmable pressure cooker) to make healthy and fast cooked meals. They cost about sixty dollars. You can find them on the Internet. There are many Instant Pot recipes books and ebooks available.

Crafting a Weekly Menu

Plan your meal menus a week in advance; then update them daily like a log. You can use an erasable planning board attached with a dry erase pen to mount on your fridge. This process will be very helpful in deciding what to cook each day, and what to buy and when.

Here are some general guidelines for menu planning:

- Consume more than 30 varieties of plant-based food (fruits, vegetables and nuts) per week.
- Consume more than 5 different types of legumes and whole grains per week.
- Reduce the amount of meat you eat. Less is better, no meat is best.
- Eat a light and early supper. It is best not to have any food after 7 p.m. For seniors, no drinks after 7 p.m.
- Drink water at room temperature before or after meals. It is best not to put ice in your water because ice cold water dampens our digestive juices and negatively affects digestion.
- Commit to eating a homemade breakfast and supper.
- Be flexible for lunch time, eating out for social events during weekends.
- When eating out, know how food was prepared, watch for freshness and wholeness, order an extra side dish of vegetables or fresh salad, watch portion size, and plan ahead to balance a rich meal out with a wholesome home-cooked meal for the next one.
- Rotate vegetables, dals, and garnishes during the week. Your mantra should be: Fresh, whole, organic.
- Sautéed vegetables can be prepared by substituting different seasonal vegetables—mix and match.
- Dal can be prepared by substituting different legumes and garnishing them differently—mix and match.
- Soups can be prepared by substituting different seasonal vegetables. Again, mix and match, and garnish them differently with seasonal herbs.
- Curry vegetables can be also be prepared by substituting different seasonal vegetables—mix and match, and learn to improvise.
- Eat fresh and avoid leftovers.

- Experiment with other cuisines such as Italian, Spanish, Mexican, Thai, etc. Get to know their herbs and spices, and store a few in your pantry, preferably whole, not ground.

Improvise with Vedic Cooking

Vedic cooking uses a small amount of healthy omega-3 oil in cooking compared to Indian cooking with fried food and spicy curries in restaurants. Using these simple principles, you can improvise recipes from other cuisines, such as Italian, Spanish, Mediterranean, Chinese, Thai, or African, and make them part of your culinary repertoire. Western cultures have used relatively fewer spices and herbs in their cooking, but they can be flavored for a more intense taste as well as creating greater health benefits using this Vedic principle.

Use the recipes provided in this book and feel free to improvise, mix and match, with different fresh seasonal vegetables as well as a variety of soups and dal.

A Word about Calories

In general, counting calories is not needed to achieve a healthy, balanced diet. However, it is important to be mindful of the portions and ingredients that you use. The following is a general framework to better understand the ratios of calories with carbohydrates, fats, and proteins. For example, if you are taking 1,500-2,000 calories in a day:

Total fat: 25%-35% of total calories

Protein: 15%-20% of total calories

Complex carbohydrates: About 40%-50% of total calories

Fiber: >30 grams in a day

Sample Weekly Menu

Here is an example of a weekly menu that can be customized to your needs and taste.

	Breakfast	Mid-morning Snack	Lunch	Afternoon Snack	Supper
Week-days	Kefir + sprouts with fermented vegetables + omelet + nuts + coffee	Fresh fruit + nuts + whole seed	At work Eat out Meat/fish (optional)	Fresh fruit + whole grain crackers + tea/ coffee	Soup + boiled veggies
Friday	Same + different vegetables for omelet	Different fruits and nuts	At work Eat out Meat/fish (optional)	Fresh fruit + whole grain crackers + tea/ coffee	Eat out (optional)
Saturday	Same + different vegetables for omelet	Different fruits and nuts	Eat out (optional)	Fresh fruit + whole grain crackers + tea/ coffee	Soup + boiled veggies
Sunday	Skip breakfast	Skip snack	Brunch Eat out (optional)	Skip snack	Khichdi

Print out your schedule and put it on your bulletin board.

Grocery List

Create a grocery list to help you keep track of what you have and what you need. Print out this simple chart and put it on your bulletin board or erasable white board. You can also make one that is customized to your particular needs.

Items	Have	Need	Remarks
Fresh fruits			
Fresh vegetables and herbs			
Fresh leafy greens			
Nuts and seeds			
Dry fruits			
Milk (non-dairy)			
Milk (organic)			
Frozen vegetables			
Spices			
Eggs, meat			
Oil			
Miscellaneous			

You don't need a recipe—just improvise. Simplify cooking with healthy spices. Recipes are like sheet music—a precise, western way of cooking. Indian music is improvised; it is impromptu, dynamic, and has sound theory behind it, yet a lot of practice is needed to excel in making it. We all can sing and enjoy; the same is true for cooking. Though I have noted a few recipes with ingredients and preparation instructions, this should be taken as a guide only. Modify as you go.

Cooking healthy food without recipes is a skill that will improve your confidence, creativity, and create relaxation. Stick to the basics of healthy cooking and don't be harsh on yourself when the dish you make does not turn out the way you expected. It's okay. You will learn the more you practice, and the gift of improvisation in cooking will become easier to master.

The recipes given in this book are all holistic and are all gluten free. They also can all be made vegan by substituting cooking oil (non-dairy), which is explained in each recipe. Be easy on salt; you can always add more later.

In Vedic cooking, crackling spices are often used as a first step in cooking. Garnishing is the finishing step. Garnishing is usually done with hot crackling spices with onions, garlic, and ginger. Or, garnish with the simple addition of fresh herbs. Both crackling and fresh herbs can be used together.

Cooking Item	Cooking Steps	Garnish (Tadka)
Dal or soup	Presoak legumes and pressure cook	Crackling spices green herbs
Sautéed vegetables or spinach	Crackling spices in a pot + vegetables slow cook with lid on (do not overcook)	Green garnish (optional)
Curry vegetables	Heat oil and fry + onion/ginger/garlic light brown + add spices and fry + add vegetables + add water cook with lid on	Garam Masala or Mustard Masala + green garnish (optional)

For details, see Chapter 10: Recipes.

Your Non-Inflammatory Pantry

For cooking non-inflammatory meals, you need to redesign your pantry and stock it with properly stored wholesome food items. Here are some helpful suggestions to get you started.

Cool Room Storage Items

Cooking oils

- Butter
- Ghee
- Mustard oil (vegan)
- Sesame oil (vegan)

Salad oils and condiments

- Apple cider vinegar
- Balsamic vinegar
- Extra virgin olive oil

Probiotics

- Yogurt starter (need to buy only once)
- Water kefir starter (need to buy only once)

Sweeteners

- Blackstrap molasses (unsulfured)
- Brown sugar
- Honey
- Jaggery

Massage and *nasya* oils

- Almond oil
- Sesame oil

Salt

- Himalayan salt
- Rock salt
- Sea salt

Spices: paste

- Tamarind paste

Spices: powder

- Asafetida (hing) powder
- Pani puri masala or chaat masala
- Turmeric

Spices: whole

- Ajwain seeds (ajwain caraway or carom)
- Kalonji (nigella seeds)
- Cilantro
- Coriander seeds
- Cumin seeds
- Curry leaves
- Dill
- Extra fine sweet fennel seeds (lucknavi), used for breath freshener
- Fennel seeds (coarse)
- Garam masala (cinnamon, black cardamom, white cardamom, cloves, bay leaves, black pepper)
- Leaf for garnishing (preferably fresh from your garden)
- Fenugreek seeds (methi)
- Mixed spices (store mixed whole in jar and grind fresh)
- Panch puran (fenugreek, ajwain, fennel, kalonji, and yellow mustard seeds)
- Whole black pepper
- Whole cloves

Spices: other cuisines

- Oregano
- Sage
- Tarragon
- Thyme

Whole grains

- Basmati rice
- Besan
- Flat rice (*poha*)

- Garbanzo flour
- Jasmine rice
- Masoor whole
- Mung beans
- Quinoa
- Whole Bengal grams
- Whole garbanzo beans
- Whole red beans
- Whole kidney beans
- Whole grain flour

Lentils and dal

- Chana dal
- Masoor dal
- Mung dal
- Toor dal

Fresh produce

- Avocados
- Fruits
- Ginger
- Lemon and limes
- Onions
- Russet potatoes
- Sweet potatoes
- Whole garlic

Nuts

- Almonds

- Brazil nuts
- Cashews
- Pistachios
- Walnuts

Dried fruits (unsulfured)

- Cranberries
- Blueberries
- Figs
- Pomegranates
- Raisins

Freeze-dried berries

- Acai
- Blackberries
- Blueberries
- Pomegranates
- Raspberries

Seeds

- Chia
- Flax
- Pumpkin

Ayurvedic medicines and other herbs

- Aloe vera leaves or lotion
- Ashwagandha powder or capsules for immunity
- Brewer's yeast
- Brahmi powder or capsules for memory tonic

- Chyawanprash for health tonic
- Moringa leaves for herbal tea
- MSM powder for body lotion/oil
- Neem powder
- Sitopaladi powder for cold/cough
- Triphala powder or capsules
- Tulsi leaves for herbal tea

What to Keep in Your Refrigerator

Fresh produce

- Carrots
- Celery
- Cilantro
- Jalapeños
- Parsley
- Raw turmeric roots
- Scallions
- Seasonal local vegetables

Note: Some of these ingredients may not be available at your regular grocer. However, they will be available in Indian grocery stores and online.

Dairy and eggs

- Cage-free eggs
- Cheeses: strong types like cheddar, feta, and pecorino
- Goat milk
- Plain full-fat yogurt
- Whole milk (organic)

Non-dairy milk

- Almond milk
- Coconut milk
- Oat milk
- Soy milk

What to Keep in Your Freezer

- Artichoke hearts
- Vegetables (cauliflower, broccoli, cut and peeled), winter squash, mixed vegetables, chopped spinach, peas, etc.)
- Fresh homegrown herbs frozen in an ice cube tray (cilantro, dill, sage, chives, curry leaves)

Planting a Vegetable Garden

Plant a vegetable garden especially for salad items and herbs. It does not take a lot of space and you can plant them in small pots.

A few of my favorites are:

- Vegetables: arugula, carrots, cherry tomatoes, chives, kale, radishes.
- Herbs: cilantro, dill, fenugreek, mint.

You can use a raised bed or a wide planter. Fill it with nitrogen rich soil with compost and organic manure. Keep it slightly moist. Four to six hours of sun is needed for most plants. Salad greens like cool temperatures, around 75°F.

Water daily, manual irrigation is best. Know the water needs of your plants, for example, mint likes more water. To spread the harvest over the season, spread out your planting, especially salad greens. Plant seeds every other week during the growing season. Pluck leafy vegetables and herbs multiple times. Cut plants an inch above the soil line; they will regrow. Visit your local farmers' market or plant nursery and talk to the growers for tips.

Here is some useful information for the following plants: aloe vera, apple or guava tree, hibiscus, Indian curry, lavender Moringa, neem, rosemary, and tulsi.

Aloe vera

Aloe vera, also known as *Ghritkumari*, soothes and reinvigorates the top layer of our skin. It contains naturally produced antibacterial and antifungal chemicals. It is anti-inflammatory and also soothes the gastrointestinal tract. You can easily grow aloe vera outdoors in Southern California and Southern Florida. It is a small cactus like plant. You can grow it indoors in a medium-sized pot, although sunny exposure is needed.

Apple or Guava

These fruits are medicinal; an apple or guava a day keeps the doctor away. Find out from your local nursery about the best kind to grow in your yard for fresh phytonutrient-rich fruits in season.

Hibiscus

Hibiscus is a hot weather plant, but it can be grown in a pot and kept inside in cooler areas. Do not overwater. Makes great tea and the blooms are lovely.

Indian Curry Plant

Curry plant is a revered culinary plant from South India, used generously in soups and cooked vegetables. It likes hot and humid temperatures. However, if you live in a cooler climate, you can also plant in pots as long as you provide enough sun and adequate water. Curry leaves are a good remedy for diarrhea. They have antibacterial and anti-inflammatory properties.

Lavender

Lavender thrives in warm weather, but French lavender is the best choice for growing in an indoor pot. It has serrated leaves, blue flowers, and is aromatic.

Lemons

Lemons are a must to keep the intestines clean, smooth, and alkaline. You can grow them indoors in a large pot. Sunny exposure and good drainage is needed.

Moringa

In Ayurveda, Moringa oleifera, known as Sahijan for ages, but known in the west just a decade ago, has multiple health benefits and nutritious value as a food. It is another "miracle tree" with anti-inflammatory and anticancer properties. It grows tall like an apple tree. You can grow Moringa outdoors in warmer climates like Southern California and Southern Florida. You can grow it indoors in a large pot in other cooler regions. Sunny exposure is needed. Visit https://neemtreefarms.com/ or https://moringafarms.com/.

Neem

Neem or margosa is an attractive broad-leaved, evergreen tree grown in India. The word "neem" is derived from the Sanskrit word *nimba*, which means "bestower of good health." In India, it has been used in many forms for ages. Indians used young twigs for brushing their teeth first thing in the morning. They ate ripe bitter sweet fruit or tender leaves as food. It is estimated that neem is present in one form or another in 75% of Ayurvedic formulations.

You can grow neem outdoors in Southern California and Southern Florida. It grows tall, so you can prune it or grow it indoors in a large pot. Sunny exposure is needed. Visit https://neemtreefarms.com/.

Rosemary

Rosemary is for all gardens—perennial or evergreen. In Ayurveda, it is also a mental tonic and improves memory. In warmer areas, it can be planted outdoors as a hedge or a garden plant. In cooler areas, you can do container gardening. Sunlight and well-drained soil are important for it to thrive.

Tulsi

Tulsi (holy basil) is the most respected plant in India. Black or purple leaf tulsi is the most beneficial. Tulsi tea made with a few leaves in hot boiling water and crushed black pepper is recommended for health and vitality. Tulsi leaves can be also used topically in facial masks for healthy skin. You can easily grow tulsi outdoors in Southern California and Southern Florida to one to three feet tall. It dies in winter so you have to replant in the spring. You can also grow it indoors in a medium-sized pot with a sunny exposure. Visit https://neemtreefarms.com/.

To get help with planting your garden, visit your local nursery and talk to the growers for planting tips. Watch a few YouTube videos to learn from the experts.

Also, visit this website for lots of great information (https://neemtreefarms.com/product-category/plants/living-plants/) for neem, Moringa, tulsi and aloe plants. They ship live plants directly to your home.

Chapter 4

Move Your Body

Exercise is a healthy and easy prescription that reduces inflammation, cleanses and detoxifies the body, and prevents disease. Movement of any kind is a simple habit. The results are positive and cumulative. Move throughout the day and it will add up to several thousand steps. When it comes to exercise, remember these three things:

1. Move, stretch, and do gentle yoga.
2. Motion is lotion.
3. Exercise is medicine.

How Much Exercise/Movement is Needed in a Week?

Approximately 150-300 minutes a week. This is only 20-40 minutes per day.

By doing 20-40 minutes of movement each day, you will gain many benefits, including:

- Being more in touch with your body.
- Boosting brain power.
- Feeling a deeper connection with your inner power.
- Feeling more peaceful.
- Improving mood.
- Increasing creativity.
- Living a longer and healthier life.

- Preventing weight gain or even reducing weight.
- Reducing belly fat and improving hip/waist ratio.
- Reducing stress.

When it comes to exercise, it is important to find the type of exercise that feels good to you. When you like the activity, you will be more likely to do it regularly. Some examples of healthy activities to increase your daily movement include:

- Biking.
- Cleaning your house.
- Jumping on a trampoline.
- Jumping rope.
- Performing yoga asanas (indoors or outdoors).
- Planting a garden.
- Playing hopscotch.
- Playing ping pong.
- Playing golf or tennis.
- Swimming.
- Taking a yoga class.
- Walking. Do this anytime. Make it a habit to park your car far away from wherever you are going and walk. Take the stairs, join a walking group. Walk in the moonlight. Walk your dog. Walk barefoot on dewy grass or sandy beach.
- Washing your car.

Note: Movement cleans the lymphatic system, adrenal glands, and skin.

Tip: You can reset your circadian body clock with a sunrise and sunset walk.

Follow the 10,000 Steps in a Day Rule

If you want to track how much you are moving each day, follow these simple steps:

1. Purchase a small pedometer.
2. Wear the pedometer on your waist 24 hours a day to monitor your steps.
3. Calibrate the gadget to monitor your steps and distance travelled. Smartphones can also be used to monitor steps and distance—check apps on your phone. You can also invest in a smart gadget called Fitbit, which is a modern pedometer you wear on your wrist and is connected wirelessly to your smartphone. Fitbit can also do sleep tracking, heart rate monitoring, and food calorie intake.
4. Gradually increase the number of steps you take daily until you get to the ideal 10,000 steps daily, if you are able. If not, do what you can and enjoy moving!

Yoga Asanas

Yoga is more than just a workout—it's a combination of four components:

1. Postures (like a Bow Pose).
2. Breathing practices.
3. Deep relaxation.
4. Meditation.

According to Harvard health, together these primary components of yoga can transform your health on many different levels.

Yoga asanas are different postures to stretch the body in concert with the breath (inhalation and exhalation). For optimal results, engage in gentle yoga for about fifteen minutes each day.

The best times to perform these yoga asanas are in the morning or evening. Do these light exercises followed by a few minutes of meditation.

This sequence is beneficial to cleanse your body and mind. These stretching exercises cleanse and lubricate your internal organs and also reduce stress and inflammation.

Beginners, Seniors, and People with Limited Mobility

As a beginner, you can choose to join a class at your local gym or yoga studio and create a sequence of postures upon consultation with your yoga teacher. Each posture has benefits for specific organs, muscles, and joints. These sequences of postures can be tailored to your personalized needs by a yoga teacher. If you are new to yoga, it is a good idea to take a gentle yoga lesson in a group class. You can find these at yoga studios, gyms, libraries, or the YMCA. You can also get DVDs or video clips on YouTube and follow along at home or in a park. Seniors or those with limited abilities can start with chair yoga—yoga asanas meant for people with less flexibility.

Yoga Asanas: Popular and Beneficial Postures

If you are pressed for time, you can start with one posture—the Sun Salutation—and perform it 3-6 times to begin. Then add a cleansing/breathing exercise, *Kapalbhati*, which is followed by deep relaxation in the Corpse Pose or *Shavasana*. Now, you are ready for meditation.

Popular yoga asanas include:

1. Bow Pose (*Dhanurasana*).
2. Bridge Pose (*Setu Bandhasana*).
3. Camel Pose (*Ustrasana*).
4. Cat Cow Pose (*Marjaryasana/Bitilasana*).
5. Child's Pose (*Balasana*).
6. Cobra Pose (*Bhujangasana*).
7. Corpse Pose (*Shavasana*).
8. Fish Pose (*Matsyasana*).
9. Half Moon Pose (*Ardha Chandrasana*).
10. Half Spinal Twist Pose (*Ardha Matsyendrasana*).

11. Hands to Feet Pose (*Padahastasana*).
12. Head to Knee Pose (*Paschimottanasana*).
13. Lion Pose (*Singhasana*).
14. Locust Pose (*Salabhasana*).
15. Plough Pose (*Halasana*).
16. Shoulder Stand Pose (*Sarvangasana*).
17. Sun Salutation (*Surya Namaskar*).
18. Triangle Pose (*Trikonasana*).

Tip: For a good fifteen minute intermediate level yoga session, visit http://www.synergy-yoga.com/ and watch their complimentary video, or see it here on YouTube: https://youtu.be/a56-vlfzutk

Note: The asanas are listed in alphabetical order for categorization only. Talk to a yoga teacher about which poses are right for you and in which order you should do them.

Bow Pose (*Dhanurasana*)

The Bow Pose is a backward bend with both the torso and legs upward while the tummy is firmly on the ground and each hand grasps the ankle of each leg. This pose gives a deep massage to your back muscles as well as stomach and pancreas.

1. Lay down on your stomach.
2. Lift your torso and legs.
3. Reach behind you to hold your ankles with both hands to create a bow shape.
4. Give a complete arch to your back.
5. Hold this position for 30-60 seconds while breathing deeply.
6. Repeat 2-3 times.

Tip: While in this position, you can rock lightly, which will sooth the vertebrae and the spine.

Bridge Pose (*Setu Bandhasana*)

The Bridge Pose is the counter pose to a Shoulder Stand. It not only stretches your body, it also massages the internal organs.

1. After coming out of Shoulder Stand Pose, keep your shoulders and head flat to the floor, bend your knees, and put your feet flat on the ground. Now lift the hips and support the waist on both sides with your hands while your elbows are resting on the floor.

Camel Pose (*Ustrasana*)

Camel Pose helps relieve back pain and strengthens your stomach, pancreas, and liver. It is similar to Bow Pose and can be done from a seated position.

1. Kneel on the floor.
2. Lift yourself, keeping your knees on the floor.
3. Place your two hands on your lower back for support, behind the navel area, and then gradually bend backward.
4. With your head back, try to move one hand at a time down to grab your toes.
5. Stay in this position for 30-60 seconds, taking 5-7 deep breaths.
6. Come out of this pose by bringing one hand at a time to support the back while moving the back forward slowly.
7. Rest in Child's Pose.

Cat Cow Pose (*Marjaryasana/Bitilasana*)

Cat Cow Pose is an excellent exercise for beginners and combines breathing with stretching. The benefits extend to internal organs, the spine, and both hand and feet muscles.

1. Position yourself on your hands and knees, facing downward, and with your toes on your yoga mat so your body resembles a table.
2. Deeply inhale and curve your back toward the ground while lifting your neck and head.

3. Pause in this position for a second.
4. Exhale deeply while bending your spine away from the ground with your neck and head facing downward.
5. Repeat this 5 times.

Child's Pose (*Balasana*)

Child's Pose is a simple child-like posture. As we age, our bodies become stiff, and this pose is ideal for relaxation. In addition, this pose provides a simple way to soothe your nervous system and keep you flexible.

1. Kneel on the floor.
2. Spread your knees wide apart.
3. Sit up straight, then lengthen your spine and bend forward, reaching your hands to the floor in front of you.
4. Let your torso lower between your thighs until your head and chin touch the ground.
5. Keep your hands on the floor.
6. Relax in this pose for 10-15 seconds.

Cobra Pose (*Bhujangasana*)

Like a cobra's raised hood, this pose requires you to raise your head and upper body while lying on your stomach. The cobra pose keeps a healthy back, relieves back pain, and corrects hunched back postures.

1. Lay down on your stomach with your legs and ankles stretched behind you.
2. Place your chin to the floor.
3. Rest your hands under your shoulders with palms down.
4. Raise your head and upper torso like a cobra while the rest of your body remains still.
5. Hold this position for a few seconds. Gradually you can increase the time you hold it, up to a minute.

6. Gradually lower your head and torso, and rest your head on your arms like a pillow on one side, then the other.
7. As you become more adept, you can make the pose more challenging by lifting your hands off the floor and stretching them behind you next to your sides.

Corpse Pose (*Shavasana*)

In yoga, at the end of each session, Corpse Pose is practiced to create complete relaxation.

1. Lay down on your back with your legs and arms completely stretched, but relaxed.
2. Start to relax your mind, since your mind is the controlling factor to relaxing each part of your body.
3. Start with relaxing your toes, then each part of your body, all the way up to your head. Send this calming message to your internal organs. A complete corpse-like relaxation is possible when you let go from your busy body/mind.

Fish Pose (*Matsyasana*)

Fish Pose removes stiffness in your neck and throat area and increases lung capacity. It is like floating on your back in water. It is also a counter pose to the Shoulder Stand Pose.

1. Lay down flat on your back with feet together.
2. Stretch your feet out and bring both hands with palms down beneath your thighs.
3. Drop your head by lifting your throat area so the back of your head is on the ground. The weight of your body is borne by your elbows, not your head.
4. Hold this position for 60-90 seconds.

5. Slowly rest your head on the ground, straighten your back, and bring your hands and legs to the Corpse Pose to relax.

Half Moon Pose (*Ardha Chandrasana*)

Half Moon pose is a standing posture that improves balance and stretches several parts of your body including: abdomen, ankles, buttocks, calves, groin, hamstrings, leg muscles, and spine. It also opens up your chest, shoulders, and torso.

1. Stand up straight with feet together.
2. Inhale and raise both arms over your head. Hold the palms together tightly with only index fingers pointing straight upward and touching each other.
3. Keeping your legs and waist fixed, bend the whole torso to the right to form a half moon shape while exhaling.
4. Stay in this position for 30-60 seconds.
5. Keeping your legs and waist fixed, bend the whole torso to the left to form a half moon shape while exhaling.
6. Stay in this position for 30-60 seconds.
7. Repeat steps 3-6 for three to four times.

Half Spinal Twist Pose (*Ardha Matsyendrasana*)

The Half Spinal Twist Pose provides a half-twist to the spine in each direction while sitting. This pose keeps the spine flexible as well as promotes healthy joints and a balanced immune system.

1. Sit up.
2. Bend your left knee toward your right hip.
3. Place your right foot on the ground up close to your left knee.
4. Keep your torso straight up, then lift your right arm to hold your right ankle.

5. Twist your upper torso and head almost 90 degrees to the left, looking behind you for 30-60 seconds.
6. Reverse your legs and do the half spinal twist in the other direction.

Hands-to-Feet Pose (*Padahastasana*)

This is a good standing pose similar to the sitting Head-to-Knee Pose (*Paschimottanasana*). This pose gives a complete stretch to your entire spine, legs, and heels. This is a great posture to invigorate your entire body, especially your nervous system.

1. Stand up straight.
2. Inhale and raise both arms over your head and with feet together, bend to touch your toes in front while exhaling.
3. Grab ahold of the back of your legs—ankle or calf—while bringing your head toward your knees, as close as you can.
4. Stay in this position for 30-60 seconds.
5. Lift your hands and upper torso slowly and then straighten your head looking toward the front.

Head-to-Knee Pose (*Paschimottanasana*)

Head-to-Knee Pose gives a complete stretch to your entire spine, legs, and heels. This is a great posture to invigorate your entire body, especially your nervous system.

1. Sit and keep your legs straight, toes flexed backward toward your body.
2. Inhale and then stretch and bend with a straight back to touch your toes with both hands.
3. Stay in this position for 30 seconds.
4. Slowly come back up to your starting position.
5. Repeat this sequence 3-5 times.

Lion Pose (*Singhasana*)

This yoga pose is designed for you to make a sound like a roar of a lion from your throat while extending your tongue out. This exercise benefits the tonsils, jaws, and ears.

1. Lie down on your back, hands to the side, palms facing up.
2. Inhale deeply and raise your head while your shoulders are still on the ground.
3. Extend your tongue out completely and open your eyes wide while holding your breath.
4. While exhaling, produce a deep throat sound of A-A-A-A-A-A.
5. Bring your head down and relax. Repeat 2-3 times.

Locust Pose (*Salabhasana*)

Locust Pose strengthens your abdominal muscles as well as your lower back while aiding internal digestion. It is the counter pose for Cobra Pose.

1. Lay down on your stomach with both hands tucked under your navel area.
2. Lift both legs together above the ground while your chin still touches the ground.
3. Keep your knees straight. The lifting can also extend up to your sacral area below the navel.
4. Hold this pose for 30-60 seconds.
5. Gradually, bring your legs back down to the ground.
6. Relax for 10-15 seconds.

Plough Pose (*Halasana*)

Plough Pose is an add-on to the Shoulder Stand Pose. In Shoulder Stand, the feet are kept vertical. The Plough Pose is done by lowering your feet backward toward your head to give more of a workout to your abdominal area.

1. After the Shoulder Stand Pose, drop both feet to the ground slowly.
2. Keeping your hands on your back, stay as close to the ground as you can. You can also lay your hands flat on the floor.
3. Hold this position for 30-60 seconds.
4. Come out gradually by reversing the process.

Shoulder Stand Pose (*Sarvangasana*)

The Shoulder Stand Pose inverted posture is beneficial to all organs and limbs. It is called *sarva*, which in Sanskrit means "all." This pose brings a rich supply of blood to your throat area and also relaxes your heart.

1. Lay flat on your back.
2. Inhale and bring both legs up vertically.
3. Keep both hands straight, close to your torso with palms down.
4. Inhale and lift your hips up while supporting them with both hands.
5. Slowly lower your back to the ground, keeping your legs vertical.
6. Hold this for 1-2 minutes.
7. Lower your legs slowly with each vertebra and relax in the Corpse Pose for a little while.

Sun Salutation (*Surya Namaskar*)

Sun Salutation is a complete warm-up yoga posture. It is made up of twelve different spinal stretches for various movements of the spinal column and organs. This one posture can provide total flexibility to the body and also help calm the breath. This can be repeated 3-6 times in a session.

1. Stand straight with feet together. Take a deep breath.
2. While exhaling, bring your hands together to your chest in the prayer position with palms pressed together.
3. While inhaling, stretch your arms over your head and arch your back.

4. While exhaling, bend forward and put your hands next to your feet. Touch the ground. Bring your head closer to your knees.
5. While inhaling, stretch your right foot back and rest your right knee on the ground. Lift your head upward.
6. Hold your breath and lift your body 6-10 inches from the ground in a plank position.
7. While exhaling, drop your knees to the ground. Lower your head to put your chin on the ground.
8. While inhaling, move your body forward and arch up. Your legs and knees remain on the ground.
9. Exhale while raising your hips and drop your head between your hands in an inverted "v" position.
10. Inhale, stretch your left foot back and rest your left knee on the ground. Lift your head upward.
11. Hold your breath and lift your body 6-10 inches from the ground in a plank position.
12. While exhaling, drop your knees to the ground, lower your head to put your chin on the ground.
13. While inhaling, move your body forward and arch up. Legs and knees remain on the ground.
14. Exhale while raising your hips and drop your head between the hands in an inverted "v" position.
15. While inhaling, stretch your arms over the head and arch your back.
16. While exhaling, bring your hands together to the chest in the prayer position with palms together.
17. Stand straight with feet together and take a deep breath.

Triangle Pose (*Trikonasana*)

This pose is an excellent overall stretching exercise to do while standing. There are many variations of it. The benefits include overall physical and mental wellness as it soothes and stimulates the internal organs.

1. Stand erect with feet apart, almost half more than your shoulder width.
2. Inhale while raising your right arm straight up, left palm touching your left thigh.
3. Stretch and bend sideways along your entire left side, feeling the stretch on the right side.
4. Stay in this position for 30-60 seconds.
5. Slowly stand back up into the starting position.
6. Repeat this sequence on the other side.

Breathing Practices

Breathing exercises are easy to do, and they are the safest and simplest way to heal the body organs by replenishing them with oxygen, also known as life force, prana, and chi.

For relaxation these simple exercises can be added to your yoga exercises, in the start with Alternate Nostril Breathing (*Anulom Vilom*) and Cleansing Breathing *Kapalbhati* (only on an empty stomach) before the final *Shavasana*, Corpse Pose.

Alternate Nostril Breathing (*Anulom Vilom*)

This popular practice of breathing alternately from each nostril cleanses the entire respiratory system and calms the mind. This can be done at any time.

1. Sit comfortably in a chair or in a cross-legged sitting position.
2. Raise your right hand to close the right nostril with your thumb.
3. Inhale slowly from the left nostril (up to a count of 8 or so) and close the left nostril with your middle finger.

4. Hold the breath for a similar count and then exhale slowly from the right nostril for a little longer, up to a count of 10.
5. Repeat the exercise on the other side by closing the left nostril, breathing in, closing the right nostril, holding the breath, and then breathing out the left nostril.
6. This completes one cycle. Repeat for 8 cycles.

Cleansing Breathing Exercise (*Kapalbhati*)

This is a cleansing practice for the whole respiratory system including the sinuses.

1. Sit comfortably in a chair or in a cross-legged sitting position.
2. Place your hands with palms upward on the crease between your thighs and your abdomen.
3. Keep your eyes open and mouth closed.
4. Contract the abdomen quickly to exhale the air from your nose. Inhalation will follow naturally.
5. Repeat this cycle. For beginners, repeat 20-40 times, intermediate 40-60 times, advanced can do 3-5 times of this cycle for 40-60 repetitions.

Learning How to Become Fall-Proof

Balance while walking, exercising, playing sports or working in the garden is a good measure of our health. It is also known as agility. Seniors are especially prone to serious injury from falling owing to lack of balance.

Some ideas to help you improve your balance, gain strength, and keep your environment safe so you can avoid falls include:

- Adding sports and activities you enjoy, like doubles tennis, walking, or golfing.
- Arranging furniture and space (closets, etc.) for traffic flow.
- Doing yoga. This will keep your joints and spine strong and flexible.

- Gardening.
- Improving your posture by sitting straight and sleeping on a hard bed.
- Improving lighting in your kitchen, study, and bathrooms.
- Installing handrails and grab bars on stairs and in your bathroom.
- Installing non-slip mats and treads especially in the bathroom, kitchen, and exercise areas.
- Keeping entry and exit areas from your house well-lit and wheelchair friendly (with sloping ramps instead of steps).
- Regularly stand up from the sitting position from the ground or yoga mat with minimal or no support. This simple habit will help build core strength and balance.
- Stretching—every movement counts.
- Walking backward a few steps slowly and carefully is also a good physical and mental exercise.

Chapter 5

Restore Yourself

The body and mind are tools that need sharpening and lubrication. The tips included in this chapter are the best ways to rejuvenate and restore your body and mind. Daily, we rest and recharge our body with sleep. We wash it clean with intermittent fasting, and sauna or Epsom salt baths. Similarly, the mind is also rejuvenated after sleep, silence, deep breathing, mindfulness, and mediation. Constantly learning new things also keeps our mind sharp. Let's delve deeper into each one of these practices to learn how they will help restore your body and mind to its optimum state.

Sleeping Well

Wellness begins through deep sleep. It is essential for rejuvenating the body and mind and keeping our immune system strong. Sleep is an interesting journey and it is a rather complex process. Our autonomic nervous system continues on as before as our organs continue to pump blood, digest food, and clean our system. We become largely unaware of our senses as we pass through sleep stages. With a good night's sleep, you feel refreshed, alert, and remain productive throughout the day. It is critically important that we get the optimal amount of sleep at the right time. Therefore, cultivating healthy sleep habits will improve your immunity and help fight chronic diseases.

Although morning people and night owls have different sleeping schedules, it is important to be regular in your sleep habits, whatever they may be. Sleep six to eight hours, preferably 9 p.m. to 5 a.m. Some individuals can do well with less, for example, five hours. Some may require more, up to nine hours. Your body will generally tell you if you need more sleep. You can gradually set your circadian clock by walking outside during sunrise and sunset. This will help you to sleep in the night and wake up early in the morning.

As we begin to sleep, we go through different sleep cycles. Initially, it takes about fifteen minutes for most of us to go to sleep. We go through five to six different sleeping cycles throughout the night, varying from light to deep sleep. You experience dreams in REM sleep, that is, the portion when you have rapid eye movement. Seven to eight hours of sleep with 20-25% REM sleep is considered good sleep on average. However, the sleep cycle is different for each of us. Infants have 80% REM sleep, which gradually decreases with age. A few smartphone apps are able to estimate sleep quality and the total hours slept based on motion and heart rate algorithms.

Here are some important sleep habits to help you create a healthy night sleep and beneficial sleep regime:

- Keep a sleep diary and discuss your sleep with your health team.
- Put an alarm on a mechanical clock a few feet away from your bed most of the weekdays. However, once a week give yourself permission to wake up without any alarm. Gradually, you may not need any wake-up alarm at all.
- Avoid overwork, intense mental work, and overeating, especially at night.
- Don't watch TV at night and turn off electronic devices one hour before going to sleep.
- Go to sleep at the same time each night.
- Keep the room dark.
- Keep the bedroom clean and adorn with inviting sheets and blankets.
- Make sure your sleeping area is well ventilated and is free of toxins and mold.
- Open windows when possible.

- Grow plants indoors to improve indoor air quality.
- Install an electronic HEPA room filter, if needed, to purify the air.
- Invest in a good quality firm mattress.
- Keep the temperature in the bedroom at night around 67-70°F and room humidity in the normal range, not too dry. It is best to wrap yourself in a blanket and not be hot while you sleep.
- Perform a ritual of washing your hands, feet, and face before bedtime.
- Listen to soothing music before going to sleep.
- Reflect on your day. Write or reflect mentally on the day lived with gratitude. Where did you go? What did you do? How aware were you in your activities and interactions? How well did you listen? Did you speak after listening completely? When did you feel connected authentically while doing an activity or sharing with people? What were the lessons? Have you cleared your mind? Learn to release anything lingering—physically and mentally—before going to sleep.
- Release and relax your body, one part at a time, going from your toes to your head. With eyes closed, feel your breath. Release the day by relaxing your body. With practice, your thoughts will slow down and your consciousness withdraws into sleep.
- Don't force sleep. If you are unable to sleep, engage in reading, writing, or meditation to calm the mind.
- Monitor your sleep every few months. You can do this on a smartphone sleep monitoring app, for example, Sleep Cycle or SleepScore. You can also enroll in the Go! To Sleep online program from Cleveland Clinic Wellness Institute and Sleep Disorders Center (see Resources).

Note: Afternoon naps may be good for some. Try them at different times and lengths of time to discover what works best for you.

If you are traveling or live in a noisy area, carry a few useful sleep-aid items:

- Blackout eye mask
- Favorite thin pillow

- Soft-foam earplugs
- White-noise machine

Forest Bathing

Forest bathing (walking in nature) can revitalize you and will help reduce your risk of all chronic diseases (heart disease, cancer, diabetes, obesity, etc.). Walking is the most natural and safe exercise, and walking in nature has beneficial effects on the mind, too. It can improve your sleep and meditation.

Sunbathing

Sunbathing in the early hours near dawn or in the late afternoon before sunset is recommended for vitamin D exposure as well as to reset your circadian clock for regulating sleep and waking hours. Appropriate levels of vitamin D prevent heart disease, diabetes, and other chronic conditions.

Most people are deprived of sunlight and have a lower level of vitamin D owing to modern indoor living. You can gaze at the very early morning sun for 5 seconds with open eyes, then shade them, rub the palms for a few seconds and palm your eyes.

Pausing and Relaxing

Our modern life is hectic and busy from the moment we get up from our bed till we go back to sleep. Our mind is continuously engaged. We need to learn to periodically disengage our body and mind to give it some rest and thus renew ourselves, making it a habit. There are many ways you can pause and relax your body, mind, and spirit.

Stretch While Working

When taking a break from a computer or desk job, stretch with both arms up then bend forward to touch your toes. Do this for about 30 seconds. Now, gradually lift yourself up with your head down, and then come to the upright sitting position. Next, move into a counter pose by clasping both hands behind your back near the lumbar region and bend backward for 30 seconds. Keep your spine erect and shoulders back. Your clasped hands help to widen your chest. This will help your posture and improve your breathing. Do this to relax at least a couple of times during the day.

Breathe Deeply

You can deepen your breathing simply by concentrating on your breath while sitting comfortably. In addition, you can inhale, hold your breath and exhale for an equal amount of time, up to a count of 10. While inhaling, watch the movement of your belly outwards and inwards while exhaling. You can gradually increase the count to 20 when you are comfortable.

Use a Sauna

Once or twice a week for 10-15 minutes, use a sauna to detoxify your body. Many gyms have dry and steam saunas. Compact infrared saunas can be installed in homes or found at some health and healing centers. Saunas have several benefits including relaxing your body, improving skin, clearing sinuses, and lowering blood pressure.

Take Epsom Salt Baths

Once a month, fill your bath with hot water and 2 cups of Epsom salt (magnesium sulfate). Soak for 20-30 minutes to relax your body and joints, and improve your skin. For an aromatic bath, add 15 drops of lavender, jasmine, or sandalwood oil, camphor, or rose water. Mix well with a capful of coconut water and pour it in the bath before your soak.

Sip Herbal Tea

Give yourself a tea break to relax. Make herbal tea of your choice and drink it hot or cold. Avoid sugar; a bit of honey is fine. Black tea or coffee in moderation is okay.

Introspect and Write in a Journal

You can make a good habit of reviewing the day and writing a few sentences, a paragraph, or a page or two about your day before going to bed. A journal can take many forms: chronological, thematic, motivational, or spiritual. Experiment and find what works for you.

Live Simply

Plain living and high thinking is an age-old wisdom in all cultures. We need to critically evaluate our material needs when we are about to spend money on acquiring big as well as small things, having less and being more.

Be Clutter Free

A clean room is calming to the mind. In a clean environment, our mind can easily focus to solve problems and create new ideas. A clean and spacious room can be safer to walk through and will prevent bodily injuries from tripping or from falling objects.

Go on Retreats

Local weekend retreats can be more relaxing and less expensive compared to a two-week vacation far away. You can explore such retreats through your local library, educational institutions, senior centers, churches, and Meet-up groups. Group retreats can provide a sense of community.

Plant a Vegetable Garden

Owning your own vegetable garden is a healthy and worthwhile hobby. You get exercise, spend time in nature, and receive fresh produce that is priceless. You also develop intimacy with your garden, watching the plants grow, bloom, bear fruit, and eventually perish.

Learn a New Sport

We can keep our mind and body agile and gain camaraderie with others by picking up a sport that we can play into our old age such as ping pong or doubles tennis.

Learn a Musical Instrument

Learning to play a few simple tunes or devotional chants on piano, guitar, or harmonium can provide hours of joy. It also exercises the mind, keeping us youthful.

Learn to Cook

Cooking something new for your family or friends can be a lot of fun and provide relaxation. Your spouse and loved ones will also appreciate this team effort in the kitchen. And, your children will learn a skill in an effortless way just by watching you.

Read a Memoir or Biography

Reading about someone you know or admire can be transformational and entertaining.

Listen to Music

You can build or record a list of your favorite songs and play them to relax.

Learn Emotional Therapy

When an external event makes us feel panicky because of a triggering event, for instance, a traffic jam, we can find calm again in the here and now. By learning and utilizing emotional therapy techniques such as Emotional Focused Therapy, a tapping technique, or a mindfulness exercise of watching our breath, we can help rebalance ourselves in times of stress or emotional upheaval.

Wear Natural Fibers

Cotton and linen in summer, and wool for winter are desirable. Natural clothing provides ventilation so our skin can breathe.

Do a Digital Detox

Internet, email, and smartphones are addictive. We are overpowered into busyness by these electronic conveniences. We do not have free time to pause and relax. This can be harmful to our health and well-being.

What can we do? Here are useful suggestions to help you create a digital detox.

Tips for a digital detox:

- Designate tech-free hours each day and week.
- Divide 24 hours into 8 hours of work, 8 hours of sleep and 8 hours of personal time, limiting the amount of technology you use in your personal time and none before sleep.
- Make your bedroom a tech-free zone.
- Periodically, stay away from smartphones.
- Put away your phone during meals.
- Turn off your phone during the night and use a conventional alarm clock.
- Work on a computer or smartphone with Wi-Fi and cellular data turned off.
- Regularly write on paper to mind map, plan, brainstorm, and doodle. Carry a small notepad and pen to be ready any time.

Chapter 6

Practice Mindfulness

Mindfulness is emptying the mind so that you can focus completely on the task at hand.

Practicing mindfulness helps to:

- Alleviate both intermittent and chronic pain.
- Calm and purify the mind.
- Enhance memory and concentration.
- Fight depression.
- Improve sleep.
- Improve your overall health with vitality.
- Increase self-awareness.
- Moderate mood swings.
- Reduce chronic inflammation.
- Reduce stress.

Our ancestors knew about the body/mind connection. Vedas emphasize daily purity of body and mind (*saucha*) practices and give us tools for purifying and calming our mind. To do this properly, we need to learn about postures for meditation and yogic breathing exercises. A silent and calm mind is our best ally. We need to train our mind and keep it calm by practicing mindfulness and meditation.

Mindfulness Practice

This mindfulness practice is designed to calm your mind and bring peaceful awareness to the task at hand.

Steps to achieve mindfulness:

1. Set a regular time to do this practice, preferably in the morning and evening.
2. Find a secluded place, indoors or outdoors.
3. Sit still.
4. Do a few rounds of the Alternate Nostril Breathing yoga exercise (*Anulom Vilom*) explained earlier. Your breath will slow down. Focus on your breath, for it is your anchor to keep you grounded in the moment.
5. Bring your focus back to the breath if your focus wavers. This is normal, so do this without any judgment.
6. Maintain peace by continually bringing your attention back to your breath. Watch your breath as an observer.
7. Watch your thoughts drift way, do not ride on them. Stay in the silence between your thoughts.
8. Be grateful for this silence and peace, and pray with an open heart.
9. Be in the silence more and more between thoughts.

This simple practice of as little as five minutes twice a day has stunning health benefits due to stress reduction. Stress is the cause of many chronic diseases. Gradually adopt this practice into your life. Become adept at doing this practice anywhere, anytime, while sitting or waiting. Please do not practice this while driving.

What is Meditation, Really?

Mindfulness is the path to enter into meditation and experience bliss. Bliss is an internal feeling of peace and joy in the present moment, and is not dependent on external circumstances. This state of being requires practice through meditation, and we can access it more easily as we become more adept at it.

Mindfulness while resting on the void between the breath is the beginning of meditation. Meditation is *not* what you think it is. Empty the mind. There is no thought in this void. There is no doing, only being. This being is everything.

Ask yourself: Who is aware when I am asleep? Who is thinking? Who is feeling? Observe: When do I become peaceful? When do I become happy? Introspect: How can I stay happy? What is the true source of happiness?

You will find that by staying in this void more and more—even while doing—you will become more calm, peaceful, and happy. This is meditation. These states are not dependent on any outer situation.

And this is who you are—really!

A few useful links for meditation are provided in the Resources section in the back of this book. However, you may want to search for a group of truth seekers (*Satsanga*) and a teacher to lead you through your daily meditation practices.

Benefits of Meditation

There are countless benefits of meditation. Here are a few most commonly experienced:

- Creates a balanced and happy life.
- Calms the mind, which through trained meditative practices is able to make good decisions in all areas of life.
- Frees the mind to keep balanced and direct activities from the center like a spinning wheel.

With a calm mind, you will be able to introspect and evaluate about your individual situation in each of these areas. Think about and evaluate your life situation. Then, color an area on the circular diagram to depict a percentage that reflects your situation. A fully colored pie chart depicts 100% of the desired state.

1. Your home
2. Your work
3. Your money
4. Your health
5. Your relationship to the self
6. Your community

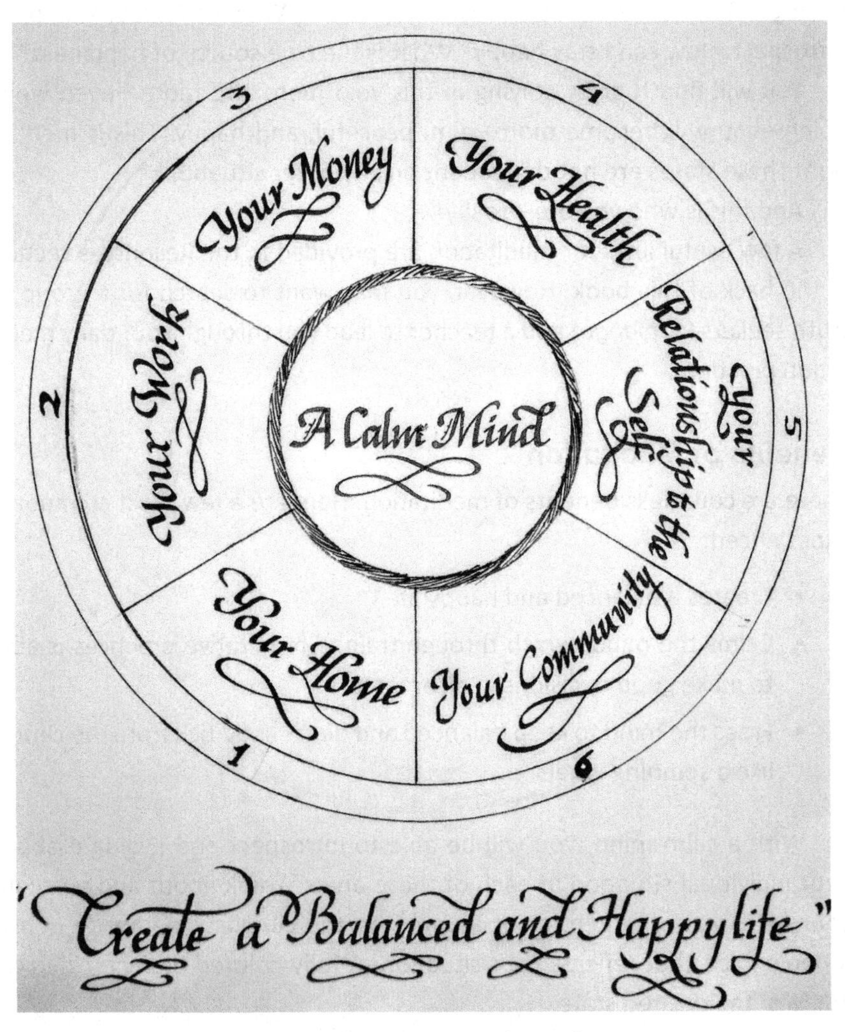

Illustration by Nawal Singh

Renewing and Connecting to Your Higher Purpose

We are each unique individuals on this planet. We are endowed with unique talents and gifts. We are happy when our talents are used to benefit others. This is the higher purpose we need to recognize, renew, and connect with. This becomes our true expression—in family, at work, or in our community. Some ideas to help you connect to your higher purpose include:

- Becoming a mentor for the younger generation—contributing to their health, education, and well-being.
- Creating a company of friends who value and support you, and likewise, in return, you value and support them.
- Staying in a college campus for vacation. Take a summer course.
- Hanging out with positive people and finding your tribe. You can do this, for instance, by joining Meetup groups that interest you.
- Being genuinely interested in people when you interact; ask them to tell you about themselves.
- Cultivating trust and love in your relationships.
- Creating physical intimacy (sex) in an authentic relationship.
- Listening before speaking.
- Catch yourself before gossiping to stop that habit.
- Joining an online commune to learn new things.
- Calling at least one friend per week.
- Admitting that you cannot change others and accept this truth with humility.
- Congratulating others on their successes or acts of bravery.
- Following the growth of young children and grandchildren, and sending them age appropriate toys.
- Spending time in nature.
- Zooming and Skyping with family and friends.
- Writing a family newsletter.

- Buying blank cards and sending loving notes or thank-you notes. People will cherish them, even after you are gone!
- Reading your favorite quotes, poems, and affirmations.
- Promoting healthy habits in your community.

One secret to well-being is to be connected intimately to yourself first and then to your community. When this is so, you can contribute to the community in a positive way and be happy.

> *"The key focus areas that I always recommend my patients pay attention to are community, spirit, emotional health, relationships, nutrition, movement, purpose, and mindset. Within these areas, we can have a dramatic influence on our immediate and future health."*
>
> **~Mark Hyman, MD**

Other things you can do to be more in balance and fulfilled in your life are:

- Read a few of your favorite quotes every day to empower you. Select those that resonate with you or create your own.
- Remind yourself of a few favorite sayings of your mom, dad, uncle, grandparents, authors, teachers, and mentors that make you feel alive, compassionate, and vibrant.

Here are a few of my favorite quotes and affirmations:

> *"Change yourself and you have done your part in changing the world."*
>
> **~Paramahansa Yogananda**

> *"What lies behind us and what lies before us are small matters compared to what lies within us."*
>
> **~Ralph Waldo Emerson**

"You were born with wings, why prefer to crawl through life?"

~Rumi

"Compassion is not a relationship between the healer and the wounded. It's a relationship between equals. Only when we know our darkness well can we be present with the darkness of others. Compassion becomes real when we recognize our shared humanity."

~Pema Chodron

"An unexamined life is not worth living."

~Socrates

"When I let go of who I am, I become who I might be."

~Lao Tzu

"A person who never made a mistake never tried anything new."

~Albert Einstein

"The ability to observe without evaluating is the highest form of intelligence."

~Jiddu Krishnamurti

Chapter 7

Build Your Health Team

Building a team for your health is an important step in creating an overall healthy life. Conventional medicine today is very effective for acute illnesses. However, it is not as effective for prevention or curing of chronic diseases. Holistic medicine, on the other hand, relies heavily on lifestyle changes—diet, exercise, etc. Holistic physicians look at the root cause of imbalance, which causes disease or inflammation. Therefore, having a team of people dedicated to helping you maintain your health and prevent disease is the optimal approach for wellness.

For example, my team consists of the following:

1. MD Internist who specializes in Geriatrics for overall conventional medicine.
2. Ayurvedic physician for digestive issues.
3. Acupuncturist for relieving pain and for disease prevention.
4. Dentist for teeth, gums, and oral microbiome health.
5. Chiropractor for structural adjustments and supplemental kinesiology testing.

I achieve balance through the combination of all of these professionals and the modalities they practice. This balance is established through a combination of prescription drugs, herbs and treatments like acupuncture and chiropractic. In addition, observation of the pulse, tongue, face, eyes, nails, and lips are subtle yet helpful indicators of any underlying imbalances.

These are examined by an Ayurvedic physician to learn what pathological processes are occurring in the body, which organs are impaired, and where *doshas* are impacted and what toxins have accumulated.

As a rule, for acute conditions, seek conventional medicine specialists first. When dealing with a chronic illness, discuss your symptoms, diagnosis, treatment, and drugs with your entire health team.

Holistic healing systems work together and not in competition with conventional medicine, but a team effort is needed. It requires conscious effort on your part, too. You need to interview your physicians, enroll them in your team and align them with your prevention and healing objectives.

How to Choose Your Primary Care Doctor

It is crucial for your well-being to have a primary care doctor who listens to you beyond your symptoms and advises you about prevention and well-being, and is not there only to prescribe drugs.

Either a Family Practice MD or Doctor of Osteopathic Medicine (DO) is a great choice for a primary care doctor since they focus on the body as a whole and work in the Internal Medicine or Family Practice division. Nurse Practitioners (NP) are often better trained for prevention than specialists. For seniors, it is wise to choose an Internist with a geriatric specialty.

The key characteristics of a good primary care doctor are that s/he:

1. Listens to you.
2. Provides timely and comprehensive lab tests, vaccinations, and diagnosis.
3. Assesses your lifestyle, diet, exercise, sleep, stress, and physical balance.
4. Partners with you in your well-being and is willing to work with other healing modalities and healthcare specialists.
5. Explains prescribed drugs including their side effects and NNT (number needing to treat).

According to Wikipedia: "The number needed to treat, NNT, is an epidemiological measure used in communicating the effectiveness of a healthcare intervention, typically a treatment with medication. The ideal NNT is 1, where everyone improves with treatment. The higher the NNT, the less effective the treatment is." (See Resources)

You can also search on the Internet to find physicians in your area who may be supported by your insurance. Here are a few ideas of where to look:

- American Academy of Anti-aging Medicine.
- American College for Advancement in Medicine.
- Paleo Physicians Network.
- Naturopathic Physicians.
- Re-Find Health.
- The Institute of Functional Medicine.
- Your health insurer and provider websites.

Be aware that many holistic doctors are not covered under insurance programs (https://www.ifm.org/). This is because insurance reimbursement is still based on symptoms and not alleviating the root cause of the disease where lifestyle is the kingpin. If you belong to a healthy empowered community, for example, a church, non-profit or an institution where you can do cost-sharing of health costs prudently, explore ways to self-insure through sharing healthcare costs. Visit the website: https://knewhealth.com/ for innovative ideas. The good news is that many of the MDs in the current conventional medicine insurance programs are changing their practice to more of an overall holistic approach for patient well-being. Do your research and find a doctor and team that work for you.

How to Become Medically Literate

1. The Internet is a great resource. However, think critically with an open mind to handle various viewpoints.

2. Get educated on microbiome, epigenetics and ACES (Adverse Childhood Experiences), and healthy lifestyles.
3. Know your ACE score: https://acestoohigh.com/.
4. Understand the cutting-edge research on how your immunity is affected by your food, including herbs and spices, exercise, mood, thoughts, feeling of gratitude and joy, and yoga/meditation. To learn more, Google these keywords: Immune Strength, Immunologic Empowerment, Immunologic Strength, Immunological Gratitude, and Psychoneuroimmunology (PNI or PIN).
5. Visit the Cleveland Clinic Wellness websites and enroll in the online courses on stress reduction, sleep, and e-coaching healthy habits. (https://shop.clevelandclinicwellness.com/collections/e-coaching)
6. Know your happiness score, how happy you are right now: http://www.pursuit-of-happiness.org/science-of-happiness/happiness-quiz/.
7. Write your own medical history from childhood including traumatic events in your life, psychological and physical injuries, accidents, parents' divorce, etc.
8. Create a chronological log of major illnesses since birth, prescription drugs used including antibiotics, smoking, and family history of major illnesses. Note diagnosis and drug treatments: antibiotics, immunosuppressants, painkillers, etc.
9. Visit your health web portal for your online medical record. Log in to your medical portal often to keep up to date.
10. View a time graph of your important medical lab data on your online portal: blood pressure, weight, cholesterol, triglyceride, A1C, glucose, vitamin D, HS-CRP, etc.
11. Outside this portal, keep a copy of every visit, medical test, and treatment you have undergone with other health practitioners out of your insurance network, for example, a holistic doctor, acupuncturist, chiropractor, a functional MD doctor, etc.
12. Talk to your pharmacist about cross medication side effects and discuss them with your MD often about possibly de-prescribing a few.

13. Put in your diary and book all your routine medical appointments together in the beginning of each year, for example, eye, dental, etc.

How to Prepare for Death

We are designed to live fully and finally. However, life is fragile and we should prepare in advance. Have any important healthcare emergency-related documents and consultations with your primary physician and loved ones so everyone communicates and is prepared. These may include Advanced Care Directives, Durable Power of Attorney, POLST (Physician Orders for Life for Life-Sustaining Treatments), your health agents, and proxies for privacy reasons. You may wish to consult your attorney.

What to Ask Your Health Team

You are an empowered patient with the most intimate knowledge about your body and mental symptoms. It is important to communicate your understanding of your health with your health team. You are the patient and the general in command. Evaluate your health team by asking yourself the following questions:

1. Do they listen to me?
2. Are they willing to work together with me?
3. Are they competent?

Your choice of who is on your team will have profound implications for your well-being.

Be sure to ask your doctors and healers how you can become an ideal patient. Find out what you can do to help them do their best job.

What Can You Do?

The most vital part of your team is you. Most people forget they have an active role in their health. Here are some things you can do as the prime member on your health team. Not only will your health care professionals appreciate your diligence and concern, doing these things will help you better maintain your overall well-being.

Make it a daily habit to observe the following aspects of your health:

- Appetite.
- Blood pressure (BP) if hypertensive or hypotensive.
- Digestive health (bowel movements, characteristics, constipation, bloating).
- Energy level during the day.
- Exercise routine.
- Heart rate variability.
- Hip/waist ratio.
- Skin/nails characteristics: color, tone, brittle, dry, skin eruptions, etc.
- Sleep quality.
- Weight.

Record each of these every day, especially the week before your visit to a member of your health team.

Observations	**Measurements**	**Remarks**
Appetite		
Blood pressure*		
Digestive health		
Energy level		
Exercise		
Heart rate variability*		
Hip/waist ratio		
Skin/nails		
Sleep quality		
Weight		

*For those with hypertension, it is important to monitor your blood pressure (BP) two times a day, preferably around breakfast and before going to sleep. Usually, BP is higher in the morning to prepare our body for our daytime activities. Monitor at home regularly, especially one week before your routine doctor visit. Find out if the BP levels are higher in the doctor's office, known as White Coat Hypertension, or it is labile, that is, it varies over a wide range during the day. This information will help your doctor in prescribing or regulating your BP medications. It is important to track your heart rate variability, that is, the gap between your resting heart rate and peak heart rate after intense activity.

Other important health markers to track include:

1. Vitamin D. Monitor your lab results and ask about which vitamin D dosage will supplement your sun exposure. Ask for sunbathing advice.
2. Monitor your HS-CRP level. Discuss inflammation with your doctor since inflammation is an indicator for many chronic conditions. Any diagnosis ending in "itis" (arthritis, sinusitis, dermatitis, etc.) means inflammation is present.
3. Colorectal health. Ask for an annual inexpensive fecal occult blood test, or a stool test. Ask whether a colonoscopy is necessary especially if you are over 70 years old.
4. Dental health. Regularly report teeth and gum health to your primary care physician. Ask your dentist to examine teeth and gums annually after a professional cleaning. Approve x-rays only if necessary for diagnostics and not on a routine basis.
5. Diabetes. Get a diabetes screening. Monitor your blood glucose with the A1C test about every six months. Discuss your weight, hip/waist ratio, diet, exercise, and stress levels with your doctors.
6. Eye health: Ask for an ophthalmological examination every couple of years, annually for seniors.
7. Prostate health: Men, monitor your PSA values. However, PSA is not a reliable marker as a prostate diagnostic test for males over 70 years of age.

8. Breast health: Women, perform a monthly self-examination and get a mammogram as needed. (See Resources)
9. Immunization. Annual flu vaccine and other booster shots as needed.
10. Medications/supplements. These may not be needed or may need to be changed.
11. Hearing. If you are experiencing hearing loss, consult your doctor to get a hearing test. How do you know if you need a hearing test? Ask your partner or friend if they have noticed a change in how you perceive sound. Note: Be very selective and alert while choosing the hearing-aid gadgets from private providers because it is generally not covered by your insurance and there are many sellers with widely varying prices.
12. Sleep. Share your sleep record or any smartphone sleep app results with your doctor.
13. Fall prevention. Older people need to be aware that injury from falling can lead to serious consequences. It is important to know ways to prevent falling and even fall proof your living quarters, especially your bathroom). Discuss this with your health team.

Another healthy and proactive thing you can do is to create a food, drink, and sleep log to have with you when you have consultations with your health team. Here is an example:

Time /Type	Food Items	Amount (one serving is the size of your fist)	Remarks
Breakfast			
Morning snack			
Lunch			
Afternoon snack			
Supper			

Time /Type	Food Items	Amount (one serving is the size of your fist)	Remarks
Other	Water		
	Tea		
	Coffee		
	Soda		
	Alcohol		

Viral Infections Including Cold, Seasonal Flu, and Pandemics

Viral infections can be transmitted to another individual, and the degree of contagion depends on the characteristic of the virus and whether people have developed enough immunity to avert it. Especially for older people, a primary care doctor may suggest available vaccines to fortify the immune system with antibodies to fight off such infections. However, vaccines are not always readily available. As a case in point, we don't have a vaccine against the common cold. The good news is that through healthy lifestyle, personal immunity can be enhanced to fight off the virus and mitigate the symptoms.

People with chronic conditions must be extra careful to isolate themselves in quarantine from viral infections. Proper precautions are advised for everyone, for example, to distance or isolate, and wear face masks to prevent sickness. The guidelines for distancing and isolation will also depend on the nature of the viral infection and susceptibility of the individual or the community as a whole. Consult a primary care doctor and adhere to their advice.

Flu-like viruses may attack the respiratory system. They can also create other serious lung conditions including pneumonia, especially in older people. When infected by a virus, check your body temperature with a thermometer and oxygen level with an oximeter. Record and communicate these readings if they are beyond the optimal range to your doctor or nurse. An oximeter is a handy, easy to use device that can be purchased for under $40. This device clips onto the tip of the finger, and displays blood oxygen levels and pulse rate within minutes.

Telemedicine

Telehealth, also known as telemedicine, is rapidly gaining in popularity and is a convenient way to consult with health professionals through videoconferencing without leaving your home. Though a physical examination may be necessary and optimum in a few cases, remote access through videoconferencing will reduce travel and provide increased comfort and safety from home.

FaceTime, Google Meet, Microsoft Teams, Skype, WhatsApp, and Zoom software apps can be easily used on your smartphone, tablet or computer device to enable the appointment with your health provider.

To make such appointments highly effective, prior digital communication with your physician or nurse through email or your provider's portal is recommended. The patient should provide the reason for the appointment, relay symptoms, and be prepared with all other vital statistics, for example, weight, height, temperature, blood pressure, oxygen level, pulse, etc. Photographs of any affected body areas, for example, a wound, sprain or inflammation may be needed during the consultation. A flashlight can be handy for remote throat examination. Prescriptions can be delivered by mail. Blood draws for lab work can even be arranged at patients' homes who don't want to drive.

Counselors and therapists use this technology, too. It is called teletherapy. These practices could potentially result in a faster diagnosis and treatment in a majority of cases. Insurance companies are reimbursing health providers to encourage these remote services.

Prescription Drugs and NNT

It is imperative you know about the prescriptions and supplements you are taking. When possible, reduce or rotate drugs and supplement with your doctor's advice. Just like prescription drugs, take supplements only when food or lifestyle changes cannot meet or replace this need. Rotating supplements and not taking them every day can be both economical and effective. Ask your doctors about it.

Use the following table to help you track what medications you are taking, why you are taking them, for how long, the dosage, and their effect.

Prescription/Supplement Drug Name and Dosage	Symptoms/ Disease and Benefits	NNT
Alluprinol	Gout: reduces uric acid	NNT: 3.8-4.5 Side effects: skin rash
Statins	Lowers risk of cardiovascular disease	NNT: 217

Ask about side effects and discuss NNT. If NNT=1, it is the most effective drug. If NNT=250, it means 1 out of 250 get the benefit from this drug.

When Should You Take an Antibiotic?

Ask your doctor. Engage in a shared dialogue about your concern that antibiotics are not effective for viral infections and they always disturb your microbiome. After taking antibiotics, it may take months to rebalance your microbiome. On the other hand, antibiotics are miracle drugs with effectiveness for treating many bacterial infections. A good physician will know when to prescribe an antibiotic and when not to.

Are You Taking Too Many Medications?

In general, adults over the age of 65 take a lot of medications. According to Medicare statistics, close to 95% of seniors take at least one drug, 70% take at least three prescription drugs per day, and 45% take five or more per day. Often, some of those pills are no longer necessary and may even be causing harm. Therefore, it is important to ask your doctor to de-prescribe any medications that you no longer need.

You May Need a Health Advocate

A health advocate is a trusted friend, caregiving professional, or a family member who accompanies you to doctor's visits, speaks up for you, and helps you to navigate through the complex healthcare and insurance system. You can contact AARP, a local senior center, or health social worker in your area for more guidance.

Ayurvedic Herbs and Supplements

In all ancient traditions, plants and herbs have been used as medicine. Ayurvedic medicines also use plants and herbs as medicine.

Some helpful herbs to promote overall health include:

- Ashwagandha: boosts immune system, known as the Indian ginseng.
- Brahmi: mental tonic, improves memory.
- Chyawanprash: overall natural multivitamin and antioxidant, rich in vitamin C.
- Sitopaladi powder: cleans and soothes respiratory tract in case of cold and cough congestion.
- Triphala powder: balances microbiome, cleans gastrointestinal tract, also used for eyewash, hair shampoo, and tooth powder.

Note: Always use these in consultation with your Ayurvedic doctor.

PART II

Homemade Healing Products

Chapter 8

Homemade Hygiene Products

Why would we bother making hygiene products at home when we can simply purchase them instead? Commercial personal hygiene products have been marketed in the last seventy years under the misconception that all germs are bad. Hence, these commercial products are laden with chemicals that create imbalance to our colonies of microbiome residing on our skin, our mouth, our eyes, our ears, our nose, and our digestive tract. Widespread knowledge of microbiome is recent and many companies are providing organic, herbal personal hygiene products that are needlessly expensive.

In the course of my own healing over the last two decades, I researched simple homemade personal hygiene products my mother used to make in India based on the Ayurvedic principles. To my amazement, I have found them very effective and easy to make. In addition, I realized these homemade products help keep the ecology of our microbiome balanced, healthy, and vibrant in different parts of our body. Replacing your bathroom supplies with oils, natural tooth powders, shampoo, and body scrubs will improve your facial skin, hair, and nails, and will save you money by replacing costly commercial supplies.

The simplest and most cost-effective personal hygiene items you can make are:

- Body deodorant spray
- Massage oil

- Body scrubs
- Eyewash solution
- Micro-abrasion facial scrubs
- Shampoos
- Tooth powder

In this section, you will learn which ingredients you need to make them along with easy instructions.

Body Deodorant Spray

Ingredients

- 1 bottle of witch hazel (or 80 proof vodka)
- Tea tree essential oil or other oils including: lavender, patchouli, rose, rosemary, or sandalwood.
- 3 oz. empty bottle with sprayer

Preparation

1. Add 2 drops of essential oil into 1 oz. of witch hazel. Shake well.
2. After shower and towel drying, spray it on your body and lightly rub with your palms. You will face the day smelling good.

Tip: Shake before each use.

Massage Oil

Ingredients

- Sesame oil is ideal in the winter and coconut oil is best in summer for the base oil.
- MSM (Methylsulfonylmethane) powder.
- Perfume oil of your choice: cypress, eucalyptus, juniper berry, lavender, oregano, sage, tea tree, thyme, frankincense, ylang-ylang).

Preparation

1. Fill an 8 oz. bottle with sesame or coconut oil.
2. Add one teaspoon of your favorite essential oil or body perfume.
3. Add one teaspoon of MSM powder.
4. Shake well before use.

Body Scrubs

Body scrubs should be applied before showering. You can apply them outdoors in the sun, weather permitting. Try sitting on a small stool in an indoor bathtub to sweep or wash after scrubbing.

Betonite Clay and Neem Powder Scrub

Ingredients

- Bentonite clay
- Neem powder
- Olive oil
- Perfume oil of your choice (optional)
- Turmeric powder

Preparation

1. Mix 5 tablespoons of bentonite clay and 5 tablespoons of neem powder. Add 1 tablespoon of turmeric powder. Store it in an empty salt container in your bathroom for future use.
2. Before applying over your body, place 3 tablespoons of this mixture in a small bowl and add 1 teaspoon of olive oil.
3. Add a few drops of aromatic oil of your preference, lavender, jasmine, rosemary, sandalwood, or tea tree, and mix thoroughly with a spoon.
4. Add just enough water to make a liquid paste.
5. Apply over your whole body with your palm in a circular and up/down motion. The mixture will become dry.

6. After five minutes, continue the motion with your palms and fingers. The flakes from the scrub will fall off, leaving the skin clean and shiny.
7. Take a lukewarm shower and rinse off.

Charoli Nut and Orange Body Scrub

Ingredients

- Aloe vera juice
- Charoli nuts (*chironji noix*)
- Dried orange peel
- Heavy cream
- Perfume oil of your choice (optional)

Preparation

1. Take 3 tablespoons each of charoli nuts (*chironji noix*) and dried orange peel and grind them in a coffee grinder. Store them in an empty container in your bathroom for future use.
2. Place half the mixture in a small bowl.
3. Add 1 teaspoon heavy cream and 1 teaspoon aloe vera juice.
4. Add a few drops of the aromatic oil of your preference: jasmine, lavender, rosemary, sandalwood, or tea tree.
5. Mix thoroughly with a spoon.
6. Add just enough water to make a liquid paste.
7. Apply over your whole body with the palm of your hand in a circular and up/down motion while it dries.
8. After 5 minutes, continue the motion with your palms and fingers. The flakes from the scrub will fall off leaving your skin clean and shiny.
9. Take a lukewarm shower and rinse off.

Black Mustard Seed and Neem Powder Scrub

Ingredients

- Neem powder
- Olive oil
- Turmeric powder
- Whole black mustard seeds
- Yellow mustard seeds
- Perfume oil of your choice (optional)

Preparation

1. Take 3 tablespoons each of black and yellow mustard seeds and grind them in coffee grinder.
2. Mix in 3 tablespoons neem powder and 1 teaspoon turmeric powder. Store the mixture in an empty container in your bathroom for future use.
3. Place 3 tablespoons of this mixture in a small bowl.
4. Add 1 teaspoon olive oil and a few drops of an aromatic oil: jasmine, lavender, rosemary, sandalwood, or tea tree, and mix it thoroughly with a spoon.
5. Add just enough water to make a liquid paste.
6. Apply over your whole body with your palms in a circular and up/down motion while it dries.
7. After 5 minutes, continue the motion with your palms and fingers. The flakes from the scrub will fall off leaving the skin clean and shiny.
8. Take a lukewarm shower and rinse off.

Red Lentil and Orange Body Scrub

Ingredients

- Aloe vera juice
- Dried orange peel
- Heavy cream
- Olive oil
- Whole red lentils
- Perfume oil of your choice (optional)

Preparation

1. Take 3 tablespoons each of red lentils and dried orange peel and grind them in a coffee grinder. Store it in an empty container in your bathroom for future use.
2. Place 3 tablespoons of this mixture in a small bowl.
3. Add 1 teaspoon each heavy cream and aloe vera juice.
4. Add a few drops of an aromatic oil of your preference: jasmine, lavender, rosemary, sandalwood, or tea tree, and mix it thoroughly with a spoon.
5. Add just enough water to make a liquid paste.
6. Apply over your whole body with your palms in a circular and up/down motion while it dries.
7. After 5 minutes, continue the motion with your palms and fingers. The flakes from the scrub will fall off leaving the skin clean and shiny.
8. Take a lukewarm shower and rinse off.

Eyewash Solution

Ingredients

- Triphala powder
- Distilled or filtered water

Preparation

1. In an 8 oz. cup, add a quarter teaspoon of triphala powder, fill it with water, stir it with a spoon for a few seconds, cover it and leave it in the bathroom cabinet for use the next day.
2. Next morning, strain the triphala water with a cotton handkerchief cloth in a cup. Use this water as the eye wash solution in the morning.
3. Repeat step 1 to refill the container for the next morning's application.

Microabrasion Facial Scrub

Ingredients

- Granular brown sugar
- Sesame oil

Preparation

1. While in the shower, combine a teaspoon of granular sugar in the palm of your hand with a teaspoon of sesame oil to create a paste.
2. Close your eyes.
3. Rub it gently and thoroughly over your face.
4. Rinse with warm water.

Neem Powder with Lemon Shampoo

Ingredients

- Neem powder
- Large lemon
- Triphala powder

Preparation

1. Mix 4 tablespoons each of neem powder and triphala powder. Store in an empty container for future use.

2. Put a couple of teaspoons (3 tablespoons for longer hair) in a bowl.
3. Cut a large lemon in half. Squeeze in enough lemon juice to create a paste.
4. Use the other lemon half as a tool to apply this Ayurvedic shampoo on your hair and scalp.
5. Leave shampoo on your head for 5 minutes, then take a shower and rinse your head with lukewarm (not hot) water.

Besan Yogurt Lemon Shampoo

Ingredients

- Besan or chickpea flour
- Yogurt or kefir
- Large lemon

Preparation

1. Store Besan in an empty container for future use in your shower.
2. Put a couple of teaspoons (3 tablespoons for long hair) in a bowl and mix it with an equal amount of yogurt or kefir to make a thick paste.
3. Cut a large lemon in half and squeeze half of the lemon into the paste.
4. Use the other lemon half as a tool to apply this homemade shampoo on the scalp and dry hair.
5. Leave it on your head for 5 minutes, then take a shower and rinse your head with lukewarm (not hot) water.

You can alternate these shampoos every other week or choose the one that works best for your hair.

Tooth Powder

Ingredients

- Baking soda

- Celtic or Himalayan salt
- Clove powder
- Neem powder
- Turmeric powder
- Sesame oil or coconut oil

Preparation

1. Mix 4 tablespoons each of baking soda, Celtic salt, clove powder, neem powder, and turmeric powder and add 4 tablespoons of oil to make a thick paste. Fill a small plastic squeeze bottle.
2. Apply to toothbrush and use like you would toothpaste.

Tip: Neem twigs have been used as a disposable toothbrush for many years in India. Cloves are also good to promote healthy gums.

Important: Pregnant or expectant mothers should avoid using neem. Neem is used as a natural pesticide.

PART III

Healthy Cooking Guidelines and Recipes

Chapter 9

Guidelines for Healthy Meals

When diet is wrong, medicine is of no use. When diet is correct, medicine is of no need.

~Ayurvedic proverb

Breakfast, lunch and supper should be taken at regular hours with at least a 12-14 hour gap between supper and breakfast the next day. You should have a good appetite before each meal. Snacking between meals is not necessary. As we age, many people reduce their intake and a few do well with just two meals a day.

A simple wholesome meal, preferably cooked or prepared at home with fresh, mainly plant-based ingredients containing fruits, vegetables, whole grains, legumes, and nuts, containing less meat and eggs, is desired. Sugar, salt, and oil should be used with discretion. Spices can be used for flavoring the food and to make it anti-inflammatory. Diet plays a vital role in maintaining our physical efficiency and overall health.

In this chapter, you will find sample menus and recipes for breakfast, lunch, and supper. Additional healthy recipes are given in the next chapter. You can improvise and customize based on the framework and guidelines provided here. You do not need to make abrupt changes to your current meals. Instead, it is best to make incremental and gradual changes and to stay in touch with your body as you go.

Generally, eat breakfast like a king or queen, lunch like a prince or princess, and dinner like a pauper.

Healthy Homemade Breakfast

Breakfast is the most important meal of the day. In fact, you are breaking your fast of 12-14 hours after your last supper. This is also the first meal of the day after you have gone through your morning personal hygiene detoxification process. Feeding the gut with prebiotics and probiotics is essential for the healthy microbiome. Prebiotics are food for the bacteria and probiotics are live food full of new bacteria.

The following tips and guidelines will help make your breakfast healthy, easy to prepare, and in alignment with ancient Ayurvedic wisdom. Do not leave home without taking this breakfast.

Breakfast Guidelines

1. Two tablespoons sprouted mung beans. You can lightly fry the sprouts in a skillet with olive oil or ghee and mix them with homemade fermented vegetables, sauerkraut, or kimchi. Rotate a different fermented vegetable each day.
2. A glass of homemade kefir. You may substitute organic cow's or goat milk, almond milk, coconut milk, soy milk, or water kefir, and rotate them or blend them differently each day. Vegans can use non-dairy or water kefir topped with one teaspoon each of freshly ground flaxseed, chia seeds, and pumpkin seeds (raw or roasted with shell on) and one teaspoon of chaat or pani puri masala for improved digestion. Alternatively, you can make a sweet kefir drink by adding a tablespoon of unsulfured blackstrap molasses. You can use buttermilk or commercial kefir if you don't want to make it at home.
3. A veggie Indian crepe/omelet made of Besan. Daily rotate a fresh vegetable selection into a one-egg omelet. Or, enjoy hot wholegrain or oatmeal cereal.

4. Two tablespoons of nuts (almonds, Brazil nuts, cashews, pine nuts, pistachios), mixed with raisins or dried berries. Rotate nuts and berries each day.
5. Coffee, herbal tea, or black tea (optional).
6. Once a week, preferably on weekends, you can squeeze a glass of fresh orange or grapefruit juice and add a teaspoon of honey.

Healthy Homemade Lunch Guidelines

1. Salad: rotate greens (arugula, kale, and spinach, while avoiding lettuce because of its low fiber content) and raw vegetables including: artichokes, black olives, carrots, celery, cucumbers, jicama, radish, and sprouted mung beans. Use natural dressings (olive oil and vinegar, lemon juice, homemade kefir ranch, or tahini).
2. Boiled or sautéed vegetables including: asparagus, broccoli, cabbage, carrots, cauliflower, peas, squash, tomatoes, and zucchini, or cooked leafy greens such as kale and spinach.
3. One entrée: mostly legume-based soup or dal. Garnish with healing spices. Eat with a piece of sourdough or whole-grain bread and butter. Rotate your lunch variety and add protein mindfully. It is best to eat less meat and enjoy mostly plant-based food.
4. One piece of dark chocolate, sesame candy, apple, dried fruit, or berries.
5. Chew a teaspoonful of homemade breath freshener after your meal.

Healthy Homemade Fresh Fruit Snack

- Avocados are better than sweet mangoes for good fat and less sugar.
- Eat oranges and tangerines with the white pith for the pectin.
- Eat local and seasonal fruits.
- One banana or apple makes one serving.

- Garden fresh and ripe is the golden rule.
- Ripe fruit has a sweet smell and bright skin.
- Ripe berries are antioxidant rich.
- Ripe pineapples have high amounts of vitamin C.
- Store fruits in a visible place at room temperature.

Healthy Homemade Supper

Eat a very light supper. Eat at least 3-4 hours before going to bed. This practice is beneficial in many ways, and it improves sleep and digestion. A 12-14 hour gap between supper and your next day breakfast, also known as intermittent fasting, gives your digestive system a nice break for recovery, repair, and replenishment of your microbiome ecology.

Supper Guidelines

1. Eat light, preferably before 7 p.m.
2. Rotate comfort food, for instance, a bowl of soup or khichdi (an Ayurvedic lentil and rice based comfort food).
3. Small green salad with natural dressing.
4. It is best not to eat yogurt in the evening. It is a probiotic food and has a cooling effect, better for breakfast or lunch.
5. Baked sweet potato or potato with skins and butter, cheese or sour cream.
6. A glass of warm water with a teaspoon of psyllium or triphala as a mild laxative usually half hour after the meal.
7. As an option, you can have a protein drink or warm milk to help you get better sleep in case you feel hungry.

Homemade Breath Freshener for after Your Meal

In Ayurveda, breath fresheners are considered a closing part of the meal. Fennel is the primary seed used in these fresheners, which improves bowel movement owing to its fiber content. It also reduces bloating. Using this after meals will freshen your breath, improve digestion, and strengthen your voice. Chewing it slowly will make your teeth, jaws, and gums healthy and strong.

Ingredients

- Fine lucknavi fennel seeds
- Freeze dried blueberries or pomegranate seeds
- Licorice candy (optional)
- Spices such as cardamom, cloves, or cinnamon (optional)

Preparation

1. Fill an empty salt or spice container with extra fine sweet fennel seeds, freeze dried blueberries, or pomegranate seeds, in equal amounts.
2. As an option, you can add a few licorice candies, which are sweet and soothing to the intestines. People suffering from heart, kidney or high blood pressure conditions should avoid taking licorice daily.
3. Store this in a cool place.
4. As an option, add a few cardamom pods, broken cloves, and a small broken cinnamon stick to the mixture to taste.
5. Add a small amount of this mixture to a small travel container (for example, an empty Tic Tac candy container). Carry this small travel container with you and take a pinch after meals (3-4 times a day, as needed). Refill daily.

Chapter 10

Recipes

The recipes included here are all vegetarian and most of them are vegan and gluten-free. In the cases when there is a dairy product, for example, cow's milk, cottage cheese, butter or ghee, it can be substituted with vegan items such as soy milk, tofu, or sesame oil. Eggs can be eliminated or substituted with gram flour in preparing omelets.

The main idea behind these recipes is that they are healthy, homemade, and contain beneficial prebiotics and probiotics. Prebiotics are food for the microbiome and probiotics are good bacteria added to the microbiome through food. Food is medicine!

Breakfast ideas given here are easy to make and not usually found in restaurants. Hence, it is important to prepare your own breakfast daily—don't leave home without it.

Lunch ideas with salads, soups, and veggies are also easy to prepare, but you may not be able to do it every day because of your work schedule. However, you should be able to dine out or buy healthy takeout meals for lunch within this framework. Of course, you can prepare meals using this recipe during weekends or holidays.

Supper ideas with comfort food such as khichdi and soups are easy to make and easily digestible. You'll love the added flavors of the herbs and spices. For soups and vegetable curries a combination of spices and herbs for garnishing are included.

Check out the light afternoon snack recipes that can substitute for supper.

A few desserts and beverages recipes are included, too.

These recipes should be used as a framework for creating healthy, non-inflammatory, primarily plant-based meals where the ingredients can be substituted based on seasonality, availability, and freshness. For example, you are encouraged to substitute zucchini for tomato in the tomato soup recipe. The same thing can be said for the vegetable curry. Improvisation is a desirable skill in cooking and is much encouraged within the given framework to prepare tasty and nutritious meals. The spices are chosen for taste as well as their non-inflammatory properties. You can customize or modify these as you gain experience.

The main idea is to eat a variety of fresh plant-based foods, more than 30 plus items in a week. This is important to build a diverse and dynamic microbiome ecology using prebiotics and probiotics that will strengthen your immune system and ward off disease.

How do we accomplish this? The recipes given here can be very useful toward this goal. At the same time, you can remain flexible to supplement your meals with other recipes or eating out.

The recipe items are labeled: dairy (D), vegan (V), and gluten-free (GF).

Note: Some recipes can be adapted to include or exclude dairy, or can be adjusted to accommodate vegan ingredients, and that is why some recipes may have both (D or V) designations.

Breakfast Recipes

Chenna Paneer

(D, GF), probiotic

Paneer, the Indian cottage cheese, has a neutral taste and it is very good for the digestive system as a probiotic. It can be eaten like cottage cheese with breakfast or can be put in cooked vegetables. My favorite is Indian sweet *sandesh*, which is easy to make. Just add sugar and a pinch of cardamom powder to paneer, mix it well like fine dough, make into thin 1/2 inch rounds, spread it on a plate and put an almond or pistachio nut in the center. Leave in the fridge for a couple of hours before serving.

Ingredients

- 2 cups of whole milk
- 1 cup of buttermilk in a spout container like a milk or tea pot

Preparation

1. Boil the milk in a thick-bottomed pan on medium heat.
2. While boiling, slowly begin adding buttermilk to the milk with the spouted pot, watching the milk curdle.
3. Stop adding buttermilk. Water will separate upon curdling. Turn off heat.
4. Strain the white fluffy product with a cheesecloth or fine sieve. Be sure to save the water because it is a good probiotic and can be used in cooking dal, soup, or curry. It can also be sipped with herbal tea.
5. After straining, wash paneer for a minute or so in gentle running water.

Serves 1-2.

Indian Crepe with Gram Flour

(D or V, GF), prebiotic

This recipe is gluten-free and can be easily adapted to be vegan by substituting the egg and using non-dairy milk and/or cooking oil.

Ingredients

- 2 tablespoons of gram flour or chickpea flour (or substitute with 1 tablespoon of gram flour plus one cage-free egg)
- 1 pinch each of ajwain (carom), mangareila (nigella seed), asafetida, and salt
- 1 tablespoon of ghee, butter, or sesame oil

- 1/2 cup of assorted vegetables: cilantro, diced tomatoes, green peas, leaf spinach, and mushrooms. Rotate a few to create diversity. Remember, your microbiomes like diversity.

Preparation

1. Mix flour thoroughly in 3-4 tablespoons of water to make a runny batter. Add spices and salt.
2. Add egg (optional) and beat it with flour.
3. Heat skillet and add ghee or butter to pan (sesame oil for vegan).
4. Pour the mix in a flat skillet. Cook it on a low heat and cover.
5. Sprinkle in vegetables. Cook on low heat and cover for 5 minutes. Serve hot.

Serves 1-2.

Fresh Yogurt Milk

(D, GF), probiotic

Yogurt is a probiotic and should be eaten fresh. Putting it in the fridge lowers the strength of probiotic. You can keep yogurt at room temperature for 6-8 hours outside the fridge for consuming with other meals.

Ingredients

- 1 cup cow's milk (homogenized whole milk is better)
- 1 tablespoon plain yogurt or yogurt starter

Preparation

1. Take a heavy-bottom pan and rinse it with water.
2. Leave a couple of tablespoons of water in the bottom so the milk will not stick to the pan upon boiling.
3. Add milk and boil.

4. Let it cool down to approximately 115°F. You can use a thermometer to check the temperature.
5. Place 1/2 cup of milk in a small bowl and add 1 tablespoon of plain yogurt.
6. Mix them together thoroughly.
7. Add this mixture back into a warm milk container.
8. Put a lid loosely on the bowl and keep it in a place slightly warmer than room temperature. Putting it in the oven (turned off) below the range top or on top of your fridge works well most of the time. In winter, you may have to preheat the oven to warm and then turn it off before putting in your yogurt bowl. After 6-8 hours, it is ready to eat.

Serves 1-2.

Fresh Non-dairy Yogurt

(D or V), probiotic

For vegan, use non-dairy yogurt or non-dairy yogurt starter.

You can use a variety of non-dairy milks including almond, cashew, coconut, oat, or soy milk. Non-dairy milk usually stays thin after fermentation. With cashew or soy milk, you may not need to add as much arrowroot or cornstarch powder. Just experiment for the right thickness. You can easily thicken by adding more arrowroot or cornstarch powder to the milk.

Ingredients

- 1 cup non-dairy milk (cashew or soy milk makes a thicker curd)
- 1 tablespoon plain yogurt or yogurt starter
- 1-2 tablespoons arrowroot or cornstarch powder to thicken

Preparation

1. Take a heavy-bottom pan and rinse it with water.
2. Leave a couple of tablespoons of water in the bottom so the milk will not stick to the pan upon boiling.

3. Add milk and boil.
4. Let it cool down to approximately 115°F. You can use a thermometer to check the temperature.
5. Place 1/2 cup milk in a small bowl and add 1 tablespoon of plain yogurt.
6. Mix them together thoroughly.
7. Add this mixture back into a warm milk container.

Put a lid loosely on the bowl and keep it in a place slightly warmer than room temperature. Putting it in the oven (turned off) below the range top or on top of your fridge works well most of the time. In winter, you may have to preheat the oven to warm and then turn it off before putting in your yogurt bowl. After 6-8 hours, it is ready to eat.

Serves 1-2.

Kefir

(D or V, GF), probiotic

This recipe is gluten-free and can be easily adapted to vegan by substituting non-dairy milk and/or cooking oil.

Kefir is fermented milk that can be easily made at home. It is a natural probiotic and unlike yogurt, requires no cooking or boiling. You can keep reusing the kefir grains contained in the tea strainer tongue simply by moving it into an empty glass and filling it with milk. You can blend the milk as you like and you can make your favorite kefir, dairy or non-dairy.

Kefir should be eaten fresh. Putting it in the fridge lowers the strength of the probiotic. You can keep kefir at room temperature for 6-8 hours to consume later. It is advisable to eat kefir for breakfast to build your healthy microbiome.

Ingredients

- 2 cups milk (cow's, goat, or non-dairy milk, such as almond, coconut, oat, or soy)
- 1 tablespoon (1 packet) of kefir starter

- Whole flaxseed
- Whole pumpkin seeds with skin
- Chaat masala or pani puri masala (optional), available in Indian grocery stores

Preparation

1. Start with a tea tongue strainer with cups to put the kefir grains inside it.
2. Place filled tea strainer in an empty glass, and then put the kefir grain powder inside the tea strainer tongue and close.
3. Fill it with milk and keep it in a secure place for 24 hours at slightly warmer than room temperature. Putting it in the oven below the range top or microwave (turned off) or on top of your fridge works well most of the time. In winter, you may have to preheat the oven to warm and then turn it off before putting your kefir glass or cup inside.
4. Next day, your milk kefir is ready to drink. Simply remove the tea tongue strainer and put it in another empty glass and fill this glass with milk and store it for the next 24 hours. This process, like a ritual, can go on forever.
5. Put 1 tablespoonful each of whole flaxseed, chia seeds, and pumpkin seeds (omega-3 rich) into a coffee grinder and grind them, then add them to your kefir before drinking it. As an option, you can also add one teaspoon of chaat masala mix or pani puri mix containing roasted coriander, cumin seeds, ginger, and salt to improve digestive efficiency.

Serves 1-2.

Tips: When you go on a short vacation, wrap the kefir starter tea tongue strainer in foil and store in your fridge for use upon your return. For longer duration, you can put it in the freezer and start to use it again after your return.

For non-dairy milk, to keep the fermented process going during winter, you may want to put a pinch of brown sugar or a date in the glass. It is also a good idea to make the first batch in cow's milk and then transfer this tea tongue strainer for the subsequent kefir making with non-dairy milk.

Yogurt kefir starter online (under $10 for 6 packets) has worked well for me for both homemade dairy and non-dairy kefir. You only need half of a packet and it can last a lifetime. You can gift the other packets to your friends and neighbors to start a kefir club like your grandmothers used to do with yogurt starters and sourdough starters. Tea tongue strainers are available online and in local stores.

Water Kefir with Berries

(GF), probiotic

This recipe is gluten-free and can be easily adapted to vegan by substituting non-dairy milk.

Water kefir is easy to make. It is a powerful probiotic drink. Water kefir contains culture sugar water and coconut water. Water kefir grains refer to appearance. They do not contain any food grains, wheat or rye. Most people prefer flavored water kefir. Therefore, you can add some fresh or dried fruit or freeze-dried berries, acai, or pomegranate for flavor and prebiotic effect. You can also use a few drops of unsulfured blackstrap molasses for sweetness.

Ingredients

- 2 cups of water, room temperature
- 1/4 cup of cane sugar
- 1 tablespoon (1 packet) of water kefir starter
- 2 tablespoons of freeze-dried berries: acai, blackberry, blueberry, pomegranate, or raspberry

Preparation

1. Pour 1 packet of water kefir grain powder inside an empty glass.
2. Pour in sugar and add berries of your choice.
3. Fill the glass with water and dissolve the remaining cane sugar.

4. Cover with a paper napkin and rubber band. Keep it in a place slightly warmer than room temperature for 24 hours. Putting it in the oven below the range top or microwave (turned off) or on top of your fridge works well most of the time. In winter, you may have to preheat the oven to warm and then turn it off before putting your kefir glass or cup inside.
5. The next day, your water kefir is ready to drink. The color will become a shade darker and will taste sweet with a slight carbonation. Simply remove 1/4 of the water kefir and put in another empty glass, fill with water and two tablespoons of freeze-dried berries, and set aside for the next 24 hours. This process, like a daily ritual, can go on forever. You do not need to add sugar the second time.

Serves 1-2.

Water kefir is a fermented drink that can be easily made at home. Unlike yogurt, it is a natural probiotic and requires no cooking or boiling. You can keep re-culturing the kefir simply by moving one-fourth of the water kefir into an empty glass and filling it again with water. You can flavor the drink as you like with freeze-dried berries.

Tips: When you go on a short vacation, store a 1/4 glass of water kefir in your fridge for use upon your return. For longer duration, you can restart the process from scratch with a new packet of kefir starter.

Real Water Kefir Grain Starter from Amazon (under $20) has worked well for me.

Sprouted Mung Beans
(V, GF), prebiotic

Germinated mung beans are rich sources of vitamins and micronutrients.

Ingredients

- 2 tablespoons of whole organic mung beans

- 1 cup water
- 15 grains of fenugreek seeds (optional)

Preparation

1. Soak 1-2 tablespoons of mung beans and fenugreek seeds (optional) in a mug filled with water for 24 hours.
2. Wash and spread them onto a large plate and cover with a soaked paper towel or cotton handkerchief for another 24 hours.
3. Beans and seeds will sprout and be ready to eat.
4. Repeat steps 1 and 2 daily to keep the process going.

Serves 1-2.

Lunch and Supper Recipes

Fermented Carrots and Beets in Mustard

(V, GF), probiotic for salads

Ingredients

- 1 cup beets sliced in small pieces 1/2 inch long
- 1/2 cup carrots sliced in small pieces 1/2 inch long
- 1-1/2 tablespoon yellow mustard seeds
- 2 teaspoons of sea salt
- 6 large lemons

Preparation

1. Put the chopped vegetables in a 16 oz. glass jar with a lid.
2. Grind mustard seeds in a coffee grinder. Add to the jar with the salt.
3. Cut the lemon peels into small strips and add them to vegetables.
4. Squeeze the lemon, straining the seeds, and add the juice to the mixture.

5. Cover with the lid and shake the jar well.
6. Put the bottle in the sun for 4-6 hours daily for 3-4 days.
7. Bring it indoors every evening before sunset. Do not refrigerate during the fermentation process.
8. Each day, shake the jar a few times and return to the sun. This fermentation process works best using natural sunlight.

Makes 16-20 servings.

You can taste the vegetables for desired doneness and refrigerate for daily use with salad or sprouted mung beans. The fermented vegetables will keep in the fridge for 12-15 days.

Fermented Radish, Ginger. and Green Pepper

(V, GF), probiotic for salads

Ingredients

- 1/2 cup ginger
- 1 cup radish
- 1/2 cup small whole mild green peppers with stems
- 6 large lemons
- 1 teaspoon ajwain
- 1 teaspoon kalonji (nigella seed)
- 2 teaspoon sea salt or Himalayan salt

Preparation

1. Chop ginger, radish, and peppers into small pieces. Put the chopped vegetables in a 16 oz. glass jar with lid.
2. Grind mustard seeds in a coffee grinder. Add to the jar with the salt.
3. Cut the peels into small strips and add them to vegetables.

4. Squeeze the lemon, straining the seeds, and add the juice to the mixture.
5. Cover with the lid and shake the jar well.
6. Put the bottle in the sun for 4-6 hours daily for 3-4 days.
7. Bring it indoors every evening before sunset. Do not refrigerate during the fermentation process.
8. Each day, shake the jar a few times and return to the sun. This fermentation process works best using natural sunlight.

Makes 16-20 servings.

You can taste the vegetables for desired doneness and refrigerate for daily use with salad or sprouted mung beans. The fermented vegetables will keep in the fridge for 12-15 days.

Fermented Sweet and Sour Cinnamon, Fenugreek, and Turmeric Chutney

(V, GF) probiotic for lunch

Ingredients

- 1/2 cup curry leaves
- 1/2 cup chopped raw turmeric
- 1 cup cinnamon sticks broken or thin one inch strips
- 1/2 cup of tamarind (imli) paste
- 1 tablespoon of fenugreek (methi) seeds, ground in a coffee grinder
- 1 teaspoon rock salt
- 1 teaspoon jaggery
- 1 teaspoon ginger powder

Preparation

1. Place all ingredients in a 16 oz. glass container.

2. Close the lid and shake vigorously. Keep in the sun for 2-3 days, shaking the jar once or twice a day. Readiness can be tested by checking on the tenderness of the cinnamon sticks. Adjust your spices by adding ingredients during curing or for the next batch.
3. Keep the jar at room temperature and use a small amount with lunch or supper as a condiment or like a pickle. Store at room temperature for one month.

Makes 40 servings.

Fermented Garlic

(V, GF), probiotic for lunch salads

Ingredients

- 2 cups of garlic cloves, quartered
- 1/2 cup balsamic vinegar
- 1/2 cup olive oil
- 1/2 cup raw turmeric
- 1 teaspoon asafetida
- 1 tablespoon of fenugreek seeds (methi), ground in a coffee grinder
- 1 tablespoon rock salt

Preparation

1. Place all ingredients in a 16 oz. glass container.
2. Close the lid and shake vigorously. Keep in the sun for 2-3 days, shaking the jar once or twice a day. Readiness can be tested by checking on tenderness of garlic cloves.
3. Keep the jar at room temperature and use a small amount with lunch or supper as a condiment or like a pickle. Store at room temperature for one month.

Makes 40 servings.

This recipe is strong in flavor. You may want to follow with the homemade breath freshener.

Sautéed Sprouted Mung Beans

(D or V, GF), prebiotic

This recipe can be easily adapted to vegan by substituting non-dairy milk and/or cooking oil.

Ingredients

- 2 cups homemade sprouted mung beans
- 1 tablespoon of extra virgin olive oil
- 3 tablespoons of butter, ghee, or sesame oil
- 2 garlic cloves, finely chopped
- 1 teaspoon garlic, finely chopped
- 1 teaspoon of green chilies, finely chopped (optional)
- 1 teaspoon of ajwain or oregano
- salt and black pepper to taste

Preparation

1. In a large skillet over medium heat, add oils and/or butter. Add oregano until it becomes light brown. Add garlic and ginger until lightly toasted.
2. Add sprouted mung beans and mix them for a minute or so.
3. Add salt, green chilies, and black pepper to taste.

Serves 6-8.

Kale or Arugula Salad with Sprouted Mung Beans

(V, GF), prebiotic

Ingredients

- 12 oz. kale (or arugula) leaves, washed, dried, and thick stems removed
- 1 cup red onion, sliced into half rings
- 1 cup apple, diced
- 1 cup sprouted mung beans
- 1/2 cup sunflower seeds
- 1/2 cup sesame seeds
- 1/3 cup freshly squeezed lemon juice
- 1/2 cup extra virgin olive oil
- 1/2 cup Braggs Liquid Aminos
- salt and pepper to taste

Preparation

1. In a toaster oven or skillet, toast sunflower seeds and sesame seeds until golden brown and fragrant. Set aside to cool.
2. In a bowl, combine lemon juice, Braggs, and 1 heaping teaspoon salt.
3. Slowly whisk in olive oil. Five minutes before serving, add onion, apple, and mung beans and set aside.
4. Tightly bunch together a large handful of kale or arugula leaves and slice into 1/4 inch ribbons. This need not be done neatly; the idea is to end up with a kind of slaw. (Recipe can be made up to this point one day ahead. Keep kale and dressing refrigerated separately.)
5. Place chopped greens in a large bowl. Sprinkle surface with browned seeds. Taste dressing and adjust spices. Pour half the dressing over the salad and toss to coat thoroughly. Serve.

Serves 4-6.

Crackling Anti-inflammatory Garnish (*Tadka*)

(D or V, GF)

This is a great standard recipe for all dal and soups. Crackling is the distinguished Vedic cooking technique in which whole or ground spices are briefly heated in a small amount of oil or ghee (clarified butter) to release their essential oils, thus making their flavor more aromatic. Each region of India can have different spices and has different terms for it, *chownk*, *baghaar*, *tadka*, etc.

A pinch of the combined recommended spices, about 1/2 teaspoon per cup of dal or soup, is all you'll need. Crackling spices are cooked at a high temperature, so use ghee, butter, or high-heat oil like sesame or coconut, to properly release the essential oils in the spices. Use a skillet or *tadka* pan, a tiny pan similar in shape to a ladle with a relatively deep well, to prevent whole spices from jumping out of the pan as they're being cooked in the sizzling oil. Butter burns easily, so use care.

While the contents of *tadka* vary from region to region, the base is more or less the same. Add 2 tablespoons of oil to the pan, then add 1/2 teaspoon each of cumin and mustard seeds. Allow the seeds to sizzle; this should take only a fraction of a minute. Be very careful because if your seeds burn, you will have to start over. Once you master basic *tadka*, you can try adding other ingredients like fresh chilies, curry leaves, garlic, onion, tomato, or powdered spices, which are added after the base *tadka* becomes aromatic.

Cumin Seed Crackling Garnish

(D or V, GF)

Ingredients

- 2 tablespoons of ghee, butter, or high-heat oil like sesame or coconut
- 1/2 teaspoon cumin seeds

To the cumin, you may add one of these options:

- 1/4 teaspoon asafetida powder

- 1/4 teaspoon ajwain (carom) plus 1/4 teaspoon asafetida powder
- 1 bay leaf
- 1 clove garlic, chopped
- 1/4 teaspoon asafetida plus 1/2 clove chopped garlic plus 2 tablespoons chopped onion
- 4 curry leaves plus 4 tablespoons diced tomatoes

Makes 4 cups.

Black Mustard Seed Based Crackling Garnish

(D or V, GF)

Ingredients

- 2 tablespoons of ghee, butter, or high-heat oil like sesame or coconut
- 1/2 teaspoon black mustard seeds

To the mustard seeds, you may add one of these options:

- 2 curry leaves
- 2 tablespoons diced tomatoes plus 2 curry leaves
- 2 tablespoons diced tomatoes plus 1/2 teaspoon chopped dill leaves

Makes 4 cups.

Five Spice Panch Puran Crackling Garnish

(D or V, GF)

Panch puran has five whole spices in equal parts: coriander, fennel, fenugreek, kalonji (nigella seed), and yellow mustard.

Ingredients

- 2 tablespoons of ghee, butter, or high-heat oil like sesame or coconut
- 1/2 teaspoon whole panch puran spices

To the mustard seeds, you may add one of these options:

- 1/4 teaspoon asafetida powder
- 1 bay leaf

Makes 4 cups.

Your Choice Crackling Garnish

(D or V, GF)

1. Heat the ghee, or sesame or coconut oil in a skillet or saucepan over medium heat.
2. Test the oil by adding just a few spice seeds to the oil; if it cracks right away oil is ready. Add the dry whole spices, for example, cumin seeds and asafetida, and as seeds crack, quickly add other fresh ingredients, for example, chopped onions, ginger, garlic, etc., and stir until pinkish brown. Add curry leaves and tomatoes and stir while frying for one minute.
3. You can add one whole dried hot red pepper to sizzle with these combos to make it spicy hot if your taste buds and stomach allow.
4. Pour the crackling garnish into cooked vegetables or soups.
5. Sprinkle with a green garnish of your choice and serve hot.

Green Garnishing Anti-inflammatory Formula

(V, GF), for dal and soups

Fresh herbs from your garden have the best flavor.

- Chives
- Cilantro leaves
- Dill leaves
- Lemon
- Mint leaves

Steamed Vegetables

(V, GF), prebiotic

Ingredients

- 2 cups leafy green vegetables: kale, swiss chard, bok choy, spinach, or cabbage
- 1 cup garbanzo bean or black gram (optional), pre-soaked 4-6 hrs.
- 2 tablespoons of garlic, chopped
- 1 teaspoon panch puran spice (or 1/2 teaspoon cumin seed, 1/2 teaspoon fenugreek seed and a pinch of asafetida powder)
- 1 tablespoon of butter, ghee, or sesame or coconut oil
- 1/2 teaspoon of salt

Preparation

1. In a skillet that has a cover, heat oil on high.
2. Fry garlic for a minute and then add the panch puran spices in high heat to crackle.
3. Stir until garlic turns light brown.
4. Add leafy greens and cover. Be careful, the water in spinach will splash in the heated oil.
5. Add beans (optional).
6. Cover and turn down to medium heat.
7. Cook for ten minutes (longer if frozen: 20 minutes).
8. Add salt and mix.

Serves 3-4.

Onion Garam Masala Veggie Curry

(D or V, GF), prebiotic

Garam masala contains these whole spices in equal parts: black cardamon, black pepper, cinnamon, cloves, and golden cardamom. Grind them in a coffee grinder before adding them for best flavor.

Ingredients

- 2 cups freshly diced mixed vegetables
- 2 tablespoons ghee, butter, or sesame oil
- 1/2 cup chopped onion
- 2 tablespoons chopped garlic
- 2 tablespoons chopped ginger
- 1 teaspoon cumin seed
- 1/4 teaspoon each coriander, cumin, and turmeric powder
- 1/4 teaspoon garam masala
- pinch of chili powder (optional)
- salt to taste

Preparation

1. Using a skillet that has a cover, heat a few tablespoons of ghee, butter, or sesame oil on high and add the cumin seed to crackle until light brown.
2. Turn down heat to medium high and add onion, garlic, and ginger. Fry until onion turns slightly brown.
3. Add coriander powder, cumin powder, turmeric powder and chili powder (optional).
4. Add vegetables and stir-fry for 2-5 minutes. Add salt to taste.
5. Add water if needed to cover the vegetables and put the lid on. Check to see if vegetables are cooked and stir to get desired consistency.

6. Garnish with garam masala and fresh cilantro leaves from your garden and serve warm.

Serves 3-4.

Garlic Mustard Veggie Curry

(D or V, GF), prebiotic

Ingredients

- 2 cups mixed vegetables, freshly diced
- 2 tablespoons ghee, butter, or sesame oil
- 4 tablespoons garlic, chopped
- 2 tablespoons ginger, chopped
- 1 teaspoon fenugreek seed
- 1/4 teaspoon each coriander powder and turmeric powder
- 1 tablespoon mustard powder
- 1/4 teaspoon dried mango powder or 1/4 twist of lemon
- pinch of chili powder (optional)
- 1 teaspoon of chopped dill or curry leaves (optional)
- a few fresh cilantro leaves
- salt to taste

Preparation

1. On high heat, crackle the fenugreek (methi) seed in a few tablespoons of ghee, butter or sesame oil until light brown.
2. Quickly add garlic and ginger, turn down to medium high heat, and fry until it turns slightly brown.
3. Turn down to medium heat and add mustard powder, coriander powder, turmeric powder, and chili powder (optional).
4. Add vegetables and stir-fry for 2-5 minutes. Add salt to taste.

5. Add water if needed to cover the vegetables, cooking with lid on. Check to see if vegetables are cooked and stir to get desired consistency.
6. Garnish with dry amchur (mango) powder or lemon twist and fresh dill or curry leaves from your garden. Serve warm.

Serves 3-4.

Khichdi

(D or V, GF), prebiotic

This khichdi recipe, an Ayurvedic comfort cleansing food for supper, is healthy and the ultimate comfort food for the digestive tract. Khichdi is prepared with rice and lentils. Every household has their own recipe for khichdi. At my home, khichdi was made with rice and moong dal. Adding a few vegetables with spicy tomato seasoning makes khichdi a complete meal. Khichdi is usually served with yogurt, pickle, and papadam.

Ingredients

- 1/4 cups moong (yellow) dal washed and split
- 1/4 cups masoor (red) dal washed and split
- 1/2 cup rice (jasmine or basmati)
- 1/2 cup mixed vegetables (can be frozen, but freshly cut green and yellow vegetables are preferred) bell peppers, broccoli, carrots, cauliflower, and zucchini, cut into 1/2 inch pieces
- 1 medium potato, peeled and cubed
- 1/2 teaspoon salt
- 1/4 teaspoon turmeric
- 1 tablespoon ghee or olive oil
- 3 cups water for cooking
- 1/4 cup peas (thawed, not frozen)

Garnish ingredients

- 1 tablespoon ghee or sesame oil
- 1/4 teaspoon cumin seeds
- pinch of asafetida powder
- 1/2 teaspoon ginger, finely shredded
- 1 tablespoon cilantro, finely chopped
- pinch of garam masala

Preparation

1. Soak lentils in cold water overnight.
2. Wash rice, moong dal, and masoor dal by changing water 3 to 4 times. Drain.
3. You can use a slow cooker or Instant Pot for faster cooking. Otherwise, use a pot with a heavy lid.
4. After coating the bottom of the pot with olive oil, add rice, dal, potatoes, salt, turmeric, and water.
5. Cook on high heat to boil, then cover and turn to low heat for 15-20 minutes.
6. Mix the khichdi well. The dal and rice should be very soft, a little mushy.
7. Add all the cut mixed vegetables, peas, and tomatoes. Add salt and additional water if you want a soupier consistency. Cook for another 15 minutes at low heat with lid on. Khichdi is ready for crackling and green garnish before serving hot.

Garnish Preparation

1. Heat the ghee or oil in a skillet over medium heat.
2. Test the oil by adding one cumin seed; if it cracks right away, oil is ready.

3. Add the cumin seeds and asafetida. As seeds crack add chopped onions and stir until pinkish brown.
4. Pour the crackling garnish into the khichdi.

Prepare the fresh green garnish. Add cilantro and garam masala and stir before serving. Consistency of the khichdi should be like runny dough or it can be liquid like soup, if preferred.

Serve khichdi hot. Complete your meal with pickle, yogurt, and papadam. As khichdi cools it will thicken.

Serves 2-3.

Yogurt or Kefir Raita with Raw Vegetables

(D, GF), probiotic for lunch (like Indian tzatziki)

Ingredients

- 1/2 cup plain yogurt
- 1 cup English hothouse cucumber, chopped and seeded
- 2 tablespoons fresh cilantro, chopped
- 2 teaspoons green onions, chopped
- 1/4 teaspoon freshly ground coriander
- 1/4 teaspoon freshly ground cumin

Preparation

1. In a bowl, mix ingredients together and serve cold with meals as a side dish.
2. You can add other raw vegetables, for example, chopped tomatoes, garden fresh zucchini, finely chopped red onions, small cubes of jicama or sprouted mung beans.
3. You can also try other cold garnishes given in this book instead of cilantro.

Serves 2-3.

Salad Dressings

(D or V, GF), probiotic

All dressing recipes serve at least 4-6 people. These recipes can be easily adapted to vegan by substituting non-dairy kefir or yogurt.

Masala Dressing

Ingredients

- 1 cup yogurt or kefir
- 1/2 teaspoon garlic powder
- 1 teaspoon onion powder
- 1/2 teaspoon freshly ground black pepper

Preparation

In a bowl, mix all ingredients together and serve cold with meals.

Chaat Dressing

Ingredients

- 1 cup yogurt or kefir
- 1 teaspoon chaat masala

Preparation

In a bowl, mix all ingredients together and serve cold with meals.

Yogic Dressing

Ingredients

- 1 tablespoon fresh lemon juice
- Freshly ground black pepper and salt to taste

Preparation

In a bowl, mix all ingredients together and serve cold with meals.

Mediterranean Dressing

Ingredients

- Olive oil
- Balsamic vinegar

Preparation

In a bowl, mix all ingredients together and serve cold with meals.

Sesame Tahini Dressing

Ingredients

- 1 tablespoon sesame seeds
- 1 tablespoon tomato paste
- 1 teaspoon tamari
- 3/4 cup yogurt or kefir

Preparation

In a bowl, mix all ingredients together and serve cold with meals.

Lentil Soup (Dal)

(D or V, GF), prebiotic

This recipe can be easily adapted to vegan by substituting non-dairy milk and/or cooking oil.

Ingredients

- 3 cups lentils (split or whole masoor or mung dal) pre-soaked overnight

- 1 zucchini, chopped (optional)
- 1 cup spinach, chopped or frozen
- 1/2 onion, finely chopped
- 3 cloves garlic, finely chopped
- 1 tablespoon of ginger, finely chopped
- 1/2 teaspoon turmeric
- 2 tablespoons butter, ghee, or olive oil
- 3 cups water
- 1 teaspoon salt
- 1/4 cup cilantro or chives, chopped
- 1 lemon

Preparation

1. In a pot with a lid, mix lentils with an equal amount of water.
2. Add chopped onion, garlic, and ginger.
3. Add turmeric and salt, then the spinach and zucchini.
4. Cook to boil and then slow cook for 90 minutes with the lid on. Alternatively, pressure cook for 20 minutes.
5. Garnish with cilantro or chives.

Serves 6-8.

Crackling garnish preferences:

- Masoor dal (red lentils): Black mustard seeds plus tomatoes and curry leaves.
- Mung dal (yellow lentils): Cumin seeds plus asafetida plus garlic and onion.
- Other dal and whole beans: Cumin seeds plus bay leaf. Sprinkle 1/4 cup of cut tomatoes and a quarter cup of fresh cilantro leaves or fresh chopped chives and serve with a slice of lemon.

Optional: Put 1 tablespoonful each of chia seeds, pumpkin seeds, and whole flaxseed into a coffee grinder to add to your dal or soup.

Cooked Spinach (Saag)

(D or V, GF), prebiotic

Rotate leafy greens: bok choy, cabbage, kale, spinach, and Swiss chard. This recipe can be easily adapted to vegan by substituting non-dairy cooking oil.

Ingredients

- 2 cups spinach, washed and chopped (1 cup frozen)
- 2 tablespoons of garlic, chopped
- 1 teaspoon panch puran spice (or 1/2 teaspoon cumin seed, 1/2 teaspoon fenugreek seed, and a pinch of asafetida powder)
- 1 tablespoon of butter, ghee or sesame oil
- 1/2 teaspoon of salt

Preparation

1. In a skillet with cover, heat oil. On high heat, fry garlic for a minute and then add the panch puran spices to crackle and turn light brown.
2. Add spinach and cover. Turn the heat down to medium and cook for 10 minutes (longer if frozen—20 minutes). Be careful because the water in spinach will splash in the heated oil.
3. Add salt and mix before serving.

Serves 3-4.

Potato Tomato Curry

(V, GF), prebiotic for lunch

Ingredients

- 15 medium potatoes
- 6 medium tomatoes
- 6 garlic cloves
- 1/2 teaspoon red chili powder
- 1 teaspoon turmeric powder
- 1 tablespoon salt
- 15-20 curry leaves (optional)
- 1 tablespoon panch puran spices (black nigella seed, cumin seed, fennel seed, fenugreek, oregano
- 1/8 teaspoon asafetida powder
- 3 tablespoon extra virgin olive oil

Preparation

1. Scrub the potatoes; red potatoes are better with thin skins.
2. Boil potatoes until they are cooked. Leaving skin on, cut potatoes with a blunt knife in four to six pieces.
3. Cut tomatoes in small pieces.
4. In a pot on low heat, add 3 teaspoons of the oil and garlic, and sauté until garlic is golden brown.
5. Add cut tomatoes, turmeric, curry leaves (optional), chili powder, and asafetida. Cook until tomatoes turn to a puree.
6. Take 2 teaspoons oil in a separate skillet and heat on medium to high. Add panch puran spices (black nigella seed, cumin seed, fennel seed, fenugreek, oregano) until seeds pop.
7. Toss this garnish mixture into the cooked puree.
8. Add potatoes to the mix and stir for 5 minutes.

9. Add 3 cups of boiled water and cook on high heat for 3-5 minutes. Stir.
10. Reduce heat to low and cook for another 10 minutes.

Serves 10-12.

Potato Zucchini Stew or Cabbage Pea Stew

(D or V, GF), prebiotic

This recipe can be easily adapted to vegan by substituting non-dairy cooking oil.

Ingredients

- 4 medium potatoes and 1 medium zucchini for Potato Zucchini Stew or
- 4 cups of cut cabbage and 1 cup peas for Cabbage Pea Stew
- 1/2 medium onion, chopped
- 2 cloves garlic, chopped
- 2 tablespoon ginger, chopped
- 1 teaspoon of garam masala powder (black cardamom, golden cardamom, cloves, cinnamon, black pepper)
- 1/2 teaspoon turmeric
- 1 tablespoon butter or ghee
- 1 teaspoon salt
- a few fresh cilantro leaves (optional)

Preparation

1. Wash, lightly scrub and cut potatoes in 6 to 8 pieces leaving skin on. Cut zucchini in 1/2 inch cubes (or cut cabbage in small pieces).
2. Finely chop or process onion and garlic in small pieces, almost like a paste.
3. In a skillet or pot with cover, heat oil and fry onions until golden brown. Add garlic and fry for 1 minute.

4. Add cut potatoes and zucchini (or cabbage and peas) in the pot. Do this carefully for water may splash in the heated oil.
5. Add turmeric powder and salt. Stir.
6. Cover with a tight lid; a heavy one is better to steam cook.
7. Cook on low to medium heat for 30 minutes.
8. Add garam masala and mix. You can add a few cilantro leaves before serving.

Serves 3-4.

Mixed Vegetable or Tomato Soup

(D or V, GF), prebiotic

This recipe can be easily adapted to vegan by substituting non-dairy cooking oil.

Ingredients

- 3 cups of cut mixed vegetables (beans, carrots, peas, potatoes, tomatoes) or 4 cups of cut tomatoes only for tomato soup
- 2 onions, finely chopped
- 1 tablespoon butter, ghee, or sesame oil
- 1/4 teaspoon of garam masala
- salt to taste

Preparation

1. In a pot with a tight lid, heat oil and then add cut vegetables (or tomatoes only) and onions. Stir-fry for 3-5 minutes.
2. Add an equal amount of water and slow cook for 60 minutes.
3. Add garam masala and salt to taste. Serve hot.

Serves 3-4.

Optional: Grind 1 tablespoonful each of whole chia seeds, flaxseed, and pumpkin seeds to add to your cooked vegetables before serving.

Rice or Quinoa Veggie (Tehri)

(D or V, GF), prebiotic

This recipe can be easily adapted to vegan by substituting non-dairy cooking oil.

Ingredients

- 1 cup rice or quinoa
- 3/4 cup peas
- 3/4 cup garbanzo beans, soaked for 4-6 hours
- 1/2 cup cauliflower, chopped
- 1 cup onion, chopped
- 3/4 cup tomatoes, chopped
- 1/2 cup wedged tomatoes
- 2 cups water
- 1 tablespoon ginger, chopped
- 1 teaspoon garlic, minced
- 1/4 teaspoon turmeric powder
- 1/2 teaspoon coriander powder
- 1/2 teaspoon garam masala
- salt to taste
- 1/2 cup tofu or paneer (optional)

Preparation

1. Stir-fry onions, garlic, and ginger in oil until light brown. Add coriander and turmeric. Stir.
2. Add chopped tomatoes. Stir until oil appears to separate from the mixture.

3. Add cauliflower and peas and rice (or quinoa) and stir for a few minutes.
4. Add water, salt, and chili powder. Bring to boil.
5. Add garam masala. Lower the heat, cover with lid, and cook for another 15-20 minutes until the rice is soft and ready to eat. To avoid making it mushy, do not stir after boiling.

Serves 4-6.

Medicinal Sautéed Bitter Melon, aka Bitter Gourd (Karela) (V, GF), prebiotic

Ingredients

- 4 bitter melons (karelas), small to medium in size
- 2 red onions, coarsely chopped
- 1 teaspoon whole cumin seeds
- 1/4 teaspoon cayenne pepper
- 1/2 teaspoon ground coriander seeds
- 1/4 teaspoon turmeric powder
- 1 tablespoon lemon juice
- 1 tablespoon mustard oil or sesame oil
- salt to taste

Preparation

1. To reduce bitterness, in warm water, add salt, lime juice and the bitter melon and soak for 15 minutes. Wash and drain bitter melon.
2. Cut the bitter melons in thin circular slices lengthwise.
3. In a skillet, add oil and heat to crackle whole cumin seeds.

4. Add onions and fry until light brown. Add the bitter melon, turmeric, coriander, and cayenne powder, and stir-fry for 15 minutes.
5. Enjoy this medicinal veggie with dal and quinoa.

Serves 3-4.

Note: This recipe is especially good for people with diabetes because bitter melon has medicinal value in controlling diabetes according to Ayurveda.

Cooked Rice or Quinoa

(D or V, GF)

Ingredients

- 1 cup rice (or quinoa)
- 2 cups water
- 1 teaspoon ghee or olive oil

Preparation

1. Take 1 cup rice (basmati or jasmine rice or quinoa) and pre-soak for 4-6 hours.
2. In a pot with lid, put rice (or quinoa) and twice the amount of water: 2 cups.
3. Add ghee or olive oil and a pinch salt.
4. Cook to boil and turn to simmer with lid on for 15-20 minutes, until water is absorbed.

Serves 3-4.

Karhi Dal

(D or V, GF), probiotic

This recipe can be easily adapted to vegan by substituting non-dairy cooking oil.

Ingredients

- 2 tablespoons Besan (chickpea gram flour)
- 1-1/2 cup yogurt
- 2 tablespoons garlic, finely chopped
- 2 tablespoons ginger, finely chopped
- spices for crackling garnish (optional)

Preparation

1. Mix 2 tablespoons of Besan in 1-1/2 cups of yogurt and a few tablespoons of water to create a soupy paste.
2. In a pot with tight lid, boil this paste with 2 cups of water.
3. Add 2 tablespoons each of chopped garlic and ginger.
4. Cook on a simmering heat for 20-30 minutes.
5. Add crackling garnish (optional) and serve with rice (or quinoa).

Serves 3-4.

Snack Recipes

Spicy Popcorn

(D or V, GF), prebiotic

Ingredients

- 3 tablespoons coconut oil or butter
- 1/3 cup of organic popcorn kernels

- 1 teaspoon chaat masala
- 1/2 teaspoon nutritional yeast (optional)

Preparation

1. Heat oil in a 3-quart pan on medium to high heat for 3-5 minutes until brown and hot.
2. Put 2 or 3 popcorn kernels into the oil and wait for the popcorn kernels to pop.
3. When it pops, add the rest of the kernels to the pot.
4. Put the lid on. Hold the pot handles and shake every few seconds until the popping stops.
5. Remove from heat and wait another 30 seconds.
6. Before serving, stir in 1/2 teaspoon of chaat masala into 1 cup of hot popcorn. Toss with salt to your taste. Nutritional yeast and grated parmesan cheese are other options.

Serves 3-4.

Spicy Corn on the Cob

(D or V, GF), prebiotic

Ingredients

- 3 cobs of corn
- 3 tablespoon coconut oil or butter

Preparation (Microwave)

1. Place the cobs of corn in the microwave with the husk still on. Microwave the corn on high setting for 3-4 minutes, depending on the microwave.
2. Grasp hot corn with an oven mitt or kitchen towel, cut cob stem and slip off the husk and silk.

3. Prepare a mixture of salt and freshly ground black pepper. Cut a lime or lemon in half and use this as an applicator to brush salt and pepper on the cob. Serve hot.

Serves 3.

Preparation (Barbecue Grill)

1. Grill corn without husk over medium-high heat, turning often, until tender for about 35 minutes.
2. Prepare a mixture of salt and freshly ground black pepper. Cut a lime or lemon in half and use this as an applicator to brush salt and pepper on the cob. Serve hot.

Serves 3.

Baked Sweet Potatoes

(V, GF), prebiotic

Ingredients

- 4 sweet potatoes
- 1 tablespoon extra virgin olive oil

Preparation

1. Preheat oven to 375°F.
2. Wash and scrub the sweet potatoes and pat dry. Leave the skin on. Poke holes with a fork and brush on oil.
3. Wrap potatoes with aluminum foil. Make sure each potato is well sealed.
4. Roast in the oven for 30 minutes.
5. Check for doneness by inserting a knife or fork into the center of the largest potato. It should be soft and uniform toward the center.

If not, cook for another few minutes and check again. Remove using your oven mitts—they're hot.

Serves 3-4.

Baked sweet potatoes make a wonderful side dish at meals. Try it for breakfast, too.

Bengal Gram or Garbanzo Bean Hummus

(V, GF), prebiotic

Ingredients

- 1 cup of whole Bengal grams, soak overnight, then rinse and drain or
- 2 cups (16 oz.) canned garbanzo beans, rinsed and drained
- 1 tablespoon lemon juice
- 1 tablespoon olive oil plus 2 drops sesame oil
- 2 cloves garlic, crushed
- 1 tablespoon ginger, finely chopped
- 1/2 teaspoon ground cumin
- 1/4 teaspoon ajwain and 1/4 teaspoon kalonji (nigella seed)
- 1/2 teaspoon salt or to taste
- a few green cilantro leaves to garnish

Preparation

1. Blend Bengal grams (or garbanzo beans), and add all ingredients (lemon juice, olive oil, garlic, ginger, spices, salt, and sesame oil) in a food processor.
2. Add water in a slow stream until the desired mixture of paste consistency is achieved.

3. Add green cilantro leaves to garnish; add a pinch of finely chopped green chilies for tanginess (optional).

Serves 3-4.

Note: Bengal grams are healthy with a low glycemic index and lots of fiber. You can store in your fridge for a few days and eat as a dip with cruciferous vegetables for a snack or as a meal.

Spiced Edamame or Peas

(V, GF), prebiotic

Ingredients

- 1 (12 ounce) package frozen shelled edamame (green soybeans) or sweet peas
- 1 tablespoon olive oil
- 1/2 teaspoon chaat masala
- salt and pepper to taste

Preparation

1. Preheat oven to 400°F.
2. Place edamame (or sweet peas) into a colander and rinse under cold water to thaw. Drain.
3. Spread the edamame beans (or sweet peas) on an oven tray. Brush with olive oil. Sprinkle chaat masala on the top. Add salt and freshly ground pepper.
4. Bake until crispy and golden, about 15 minutes.

Serves 3-4.

Roasted Flat Rice and Peas (*Poha Mattar*)

(V, GF), prebiotic

Ingredients

- 1-1/2 cups flat rice (*poha*)
- 1/2 cup frozen green peas (*mattar*) rinsed, thawed, and drained
- 1 tablespoon sesame oil
- 1 teaspoon ginger, finely chopped
- 1 teaspoon whole cumin seeds
- 1/2 teaspoon whole ground black pepper
- 1 pinch of asafetida powder
- 1/3 cup fresh coriander leaves, chopped (optional)

Preparation

1. Put flat rice in a strainer or colander, rinse and drain.
2. Heat oil in a skillet.
3. Crackle cumin seeds in the heated oil. Add finely chopped ginger and sauté for a minute.
4. Add green peas and mix well with the remaining ingredients. Salt to taste.
5. Cover the pan with lid and cook for 5 minutes until peas are cooked.
6. Add freshly ground black pepper and 1 pinch asafetida.
7. Mix well, then add flat rice (*poha*), gently mix and cook for 2-3 minutes with lid on.

Serves 3-4.

You can add 1/2 to 1 teaspoon lemon juice and garnish with fresh cilantro before serving.

Besan Pakoras

(V, GF), prebiotic

Great for snacks or as an appetizer with soup.

Ingredients

- 1 cup cruciferous vegetables cut in bite-sized pieces
- 4 tablespoons chickpea flour (Besan or chickpea flour)
- 2 tablespoons rice flour or gluten-free flour
- 4 tablespoons onions, finely chopped
- 1-1/2 tablespoons garlic, finely chopped or garlic paste
- 2 tablespoons fresh cilantro, chopped
- 4 tablespoons of extra virgin olive oil
- salt to taste

Preparation

1. Combine in a bowl and mix together salt, spices, and Besan.
2. Add oil and water (as needed) to make a batter-like paste.
3. Immerse vegetables and coat with batter.
4. Drop scoops of the mixture on parchment lined baking sheet. Spray oil on top.
5. Bake until golden brown at 400°F.
6. Cool and serve with sauce or pickle of your choice or fermented vegetables, for example, sauerkraut or kimchi.

Serves 4-6.

Beverage and Dessert Recipes

Herbal Teas

(V, GF), an anti-inflammatory drink

Ingredients

- 2 cups water
- 8-10 leaves of Moringa, tulsi, hibiscus, or lavender flower
- 1/2 teaspoon freshly chopped ginger or ginger powder (optional)
- 1/2 teaspoon cloves (optional)
- 1/2 teaspoon turmeric (optional)
- 1/2 teaspoon thyme (optional)
- 1-2 teaspoon of honey (optional)
- twist of lemon

Preparation

1. In 2 cups of boiling water, cook leaves for 2-3 minutes. Pour in a cup and garnish as desired from the ingredients above.
2. Serve with honey and a twist of lemon and sip leisurely.

Serves 1-2.

Manjistha tea is very good for improving digestion. It can be made with whole spices (cumin, fennel, coriander, and manjistha leaves). After cooking in the boiling water for 3-5 minutes, drain the spices and serve this tea with added ingredients as you desire.

Moringa and tulsi tea are anti-inflammatory, anti-cancer, and they improve gut health.

Hibiscus tea is good for blood pressure, diabetes, and cholesterol.

Lavender tea is good for relaxation and detoxification.

Cucumber Mint Summer Lassi Drink

(D or V, GF), probiotic

Lassi is a healthful yogurt-based drink popular throughout India. Mint and ginger give it a tangy and refreshing taste. Mint lassi is a great compliment to any meal, especially during summer.

This recipe can be easily adapted to vegan by substituting non-dairy yogurt. For example, you can replace yogurt with almond milk, but do not add additional water.

Ingredients

- 2 cups cucumber, finely chopped
- 1/2 cup yogurt or kefir (homemade is best)
- 1 tablespoon of pani puri or chaat masala
- a few mint leaves (from your garden is best)
- 1 teaspoon ginger, finely chopped (optional)
- 1/2 cup of ice cubes

Preparation

1. Blend cucumber, yogurt or kefir, and spice powder.
2. In two glasses, split ice cubes and toss in a few mint leaves.
3. Pour the mixture over ice and serve.

Serves 1-2.

Salted Mint Lassi Drink

(D or V, GF), probiotic

This recipe can be easily adapted to vegan by substituting non-dairy yogurt. For example, you can replace yogurt with almond milk, but do not add additional water.

Ingredients

- 2 cups yogurt (homemade is best)
- 2 cups water
- 1 tablespoon of pani puri or chaat masala
- a few mint leaves (from your garden is best)
- 1/2 cup of ice cubes

Preparation

1. Blend yogurt, water, sugar, mint leaves, and spice powder together.
2. In two glasses, split ice cubes and toss in a few mint leaves.
3. Pour the mixture over ice and serve.

Serves 1-2.

Sweet Lassi Drink

(D or V, GF), probiotic

This recipe can be easily adapted to vegan by substituting non-dairy yogurt. For example, you can replace yogurt with almond milk, but do not add additional water.

Ingredients

- 2 cups yogurt (homemade is best)
- 2 cups water
- 2 tablespoons sugar
- 1 teaspoon rose water
- 1/2 teaspoon of cardamom powder, freshly crushed
- 1/2 cup of ice cubes

Preparation

1. In two glasses, split ice cubes and pour rose water half and half.
2. Blend yogurt, water, sugar, and cardamom powder together to make it thick and a bit frothy.
3. Pour the mix over ice in the two glasses and serve.

Serves 2.

Variations

Try adding 1 cup of mango or two cups of strawberry. Garnish with fresh mint leaves, leaving out the cardamom or rose water. Add sugar to taste.

Shrikhand

(D, GF), probiotic

Shrikhand is a classic dessert of Western India. Plain yogurt is transformed into an aromatic delicacy flavored with saffron and cardamom.

Ingredients

- 4 cups of yogurt (homemade is best)
- 3/4 cup of sugar, adjust to taste
- 1/4 teaspoon crushed cardamom
- 1 tablespoon sliced almonds
- 1 tablespoon sliced pistachios

Preparation

1. Drain the yogurt in muslin or cheesecloth over a strainer. Collect the water by placing a bowl underneath. This water is a good probiotic for drinking or making soups, dal, or curry.

2. Press gently to squeeze the excess water from yogurt and place the yogurt with the strainer and bowl into the refrigerator for 4-6 hours to make yogurt very thick.
3. Add sugar and cardamom powder to yogurt and mix it like a fine dough with a mixer or food processor.
4. Knead well until sugar dissolves.
5. Add almonds and pistachios to the yogurt mix. Refrigerate and serve cold.

Serves 4-6.

PART IV

Living Your Healthiest Life

Chapter 11

Applying this Wisdom

Health is above wealth and wise people know this. The earlier we come to realize this wisdom, the sooner we reap the rewards. However, it is never too late to follow these tips. Our body is an amazing machine. It is much more complex than an automobile. Often, we do not take care of our body. Many of us, especially young adults, take our body for granted. Unlike a car, we do not clean the air intake filter or food intake filter, nor wash and wax it from outside or vacuum it from inside. We do not check the nutrition octane level of food that we consume.

Interestingly, we do not turn off the ignition when we park ourselves at our destination. We do not rest our mind, we keep it idling with worries and repetitive or negative thoughts, and we stay awake when we should be sleeping.

The most amazing news is that our human equipment is infinitely intelligent. Our body and mind regenerates and heals itself. It can repair itself and even forgives our past mistakes as we make amends at any age.

So, let us engage ourselves in the pursuit of health that is essential for our happiness. The following is a checklist of important healthy habits to help you on your journey.

List of Important Good Habits for Well-Being

Ask yourself the following questions at the end of the day to help you determine your progress on adopting and maintaining these good habits for well-being. Small changes in your lifestyle today can bring large dividends for you later on.

Today did you:

- Perform your daily personal detoxification: oil pulling, neti, *nasya*, eyewash, tooth powder brushing, tongue scraping, etc.?
- Have a regular and good bowel movement?
- Give yourself a head-to-toe massage?
- Eat at least six servings of fruits and vegetables?
- Consume a dairy or non-dairy probiotic like kefir or yogurt? Did you make it yourself?
- Eat your own sprouted mung beans for breakfast?
- Eat a spoonful of fermented vegetables and spices with sprouts or a salad?
- Eat a tablespoonful of freshly ground flaxseed, pumpkin seeds, and chia seeds?
- Eat a few nuts and seeds?
- Eat dark, green leafy vegetables?
- Eat legume-based soups or meals?
- Eat mostly alkaline, low glycemic index foods?
- Cook or make at least one meal yourself?
- Drink water at room temperature between meals as your main beverage?
- Avoid soda, artificial sweeteners, and excessive sugar?
- Avoid processed food?
- Eat a light supper?
- Have a gap of at least twelve hours between supper and breakfast?
- Walk a few thousands steps?
- Do yoga for ten minutes or more?
- Meditate for ten minutes or more?

- Sleep well last night (7-9 hours)?
- Feel grateful for at least three things?
- Feel excited upon waking up?
- Feel connected with a loved one?
- Feel connected with nature?

And did you:

- Eat a variety of fresh vegetables and ripe fruits throughout the week (about 25-30)?
- Recently consult with an Integrative MD or Naturopath for the prevention of diseases?

Chapter 12

May You BE Healthy

When I thought of writing this book, like many authors, I often asked myself these three questions:

1. Why am I writing this book?
2. Who will read this book?
3. Can readers benefit from reading this book?

I have been a patient with a host of chronic diseases most of my adult life. I have experienced a heart attack, congestive heart failure, and implantation of an AICD/Pacemaker. Today, my heart is healthy and as a result of this fact, the AICD/Pacemaker has been disabled. Now that my chronic conditions are greatly relieved, at the age of 72 years, I am able to lead the healthiest part of my life. My fervent desire is that people much younger than me will read this book to get the maximum benefit throughout their lives. I wish to be of help and to empower others, which is why I offer this book to you, dear reader, whomever you may be.

I kept my grandchildren in mind, all under six years old today, as readers, and hope this book will help them retain their health as they grow up. Of course, I also hope that my grandchildren will start the Ayurvedic *dinacharya* routine as early as possible with training and guidance from their parents.

I believe my readers will benefit from the age-old Ayurvedic wisdom and practices that are reinforced by the modern discovery of the microbiome.

A few MDs have called this a milestone, the missing organ they now know about. Current research papers claim that 90% of chronic diseases can be prevented or relieved through lifestyle. Clearly, by changing our lifestyle, we can triumph over chronic diseases.

According to Ayurveda, "All disease begins in the gut." It is amazing the ancient rishis of India knew this. My beloved sister, Vidya Didi, and my brother, Bharatji, lived exemplary lives using these principles. They inspired me and motivated me to continue to heal and share all I have learned. Rishis of India have affirmed, "May we all be healthy and disease-free." Hence, this book is dedicated to them.

May this truth empower each one of us to now live our healthiest life. May you BE healthy!

Chapter 13

Resources

Introduction

Articles to Read

"The human microbiome: why our microbes could be key to our health," *The Guardian*, March 26, 2018, https://www.theguardian.com/news/2018/mar/26/the-human-microbiome-why-our-microbes-could-be-key-to-our-health)

"Top 10 Health Concerns of Baby Boomers," Scripps, July 27, 2018, https://www.scripps.org/news_items/5475-top-health-concerns-of-baby-boomers

Meggs.,M.D.,WilliamJoel,andSvec,Carol,*TheInflammationCure*,2005, https://www.amazon.com/Inflammation-Cure-Reversing-arthritis-Alzheimers/dp/0071438718/ref=sr_1_fkmr1_1?keywords=Inflammation+Cure%2C+2003+meggs&qid=1582844111&s=books&sr=1-1-fkmr1

Chapter 1: Daily and Natural Detoxification

Books to Read

Guarneri, M.D., Mimi. *108 Pearls to Awaken Your Healing Potential: A Cardiologist Translates the Science of Health and Healing into Practice*. Hay House, 2017, https://www.amazon.com/Pearls-Awaken-Your-Healing-Potential/dp/1401945775

Nakazawa, Donna. *The Last Best Cure: My Quest to Awaken the Healing Parts of My Brain, and Get My Body, My Joy, and My Life.* Avery, 2013, https://www.amazon.com/Last-Best-Cure-Awaken-Healing/dp/159463128X/ref=sr_1_1?keywords=The+last+best+cure&qid=1582256102&s=books&sr=1-1

Telpner, Meghan. *UnDiet: Eat Your Way to Vibrant Health.* McClelland and Stewart, 2013, https://amazon.com/UnDiet-by-Meghan-Telpner-2013-01-25/dp/B019TLB9YQ

Ornish, M.D., Dean, and Ornish, Anne. *Undo It!: How Simple Lifestyle Changes Can Reverse Most Chronic Diseases.* Ballantine, 2019, https://amazon.com/Undo-Lifestyle-Changes-Reverse-Diseases/dp/052547997X

Health Literacy

Say-Ah Health Literacy website provides the ability to find and understand basic health and medical information: http://say-ah.org/about-health-literacy/frequently-asked-questions

Education on Healthy Habits

American College of Lifestyle Medicine: https://www.lifestylemedicine.org

US Department of Health and Human Services, My Health Finder: https://health.gov/myhealthfinder

Centers for Disease Control: https://www.cdc.gov/

Livestrong: https://www.livestrong.org/

National Institutes of Health: https://www.nih.gov/

Rose Caiola embarked on a journey to uncover the roots of well-being to create harmony and balance in both her personal and professional life. Hence, the website Rewire Me was born: https://www.rewireme.com/

The Mayo Clinic: https://www.mayoclinic.org/

Vitality: http://vitality.com/

WebMD: https://www.webmd.com/

Well: at the intersection of health, green living, and conscious commerce: https://www.well.org/

Books to Read

Bhattacharya, Bhaswati. *Everyday Ayurveda: Daily Habits That Can Change Your Life in a Day*. Ebury Press, 2015, https://www.amazon.com/Everyday-Ayurveda-Daily-Habits-Change-ebook/dp/B015O6BC4C

Helpful Products

Personal Detox Kit (Eye Wash, Neti Pot, and Tongue Cleaner): https://smile.amazon.com/gp/product/B0761VG83G/ref=ppx_yo_dt_b_asin_title_o00__o00_s00?ie=UTF8&psc=1

Quick Drying Microfiber Bath Towel: https://www.amazon.com/Rainleaf-Microfiber-Towel-Inches-Green/dp/B01A4ZXVOM/ref=sr_1_1_sspa?ie=UTF8&qid=1550511933&sr=8-1-spons&keywords=rainleaf+towel&psc=1

Quick Drying Cotton Bath Towel: https://www.amazon.com/Craftbot-Towels-Lightweight-Cotton-Inches/dp/B07KLRYK22/ref=sr_1_12_sspa?ie=UTF8&qid=1550512157&sr=8-12-spons&keywords=handloom+towel&psc=1

Chapters 2 &3: Food is Medicine and Healthy Food Habits

Chia Seeds

https://smile.amazon.com/gp/product/B00OZYNGUS/ref=ppx_yo_dt_b_asin_title_o02__o00_s00?ie=UTF8&th=1

Fermented Foods

Farm Ferments: https://farmferments.com/

Fermented Foods List (International)

Wikipedia list: https://en.m.wikipedia.org/wiki/List_of_fermented_foods

The Fermentationist: https://fermentationist.com/

Flaxseed

Non-GMO flaxseed: https://smile.amazon.com/Organic-Golden-Flax-seed-Non-GMO-Food/dp/B01M6WOIAG/ref=sr_1_3_s_it?s=grocery &ie=UTF8&qid=1550685299&sr=1-3-spons&keywords=flaxseed%2B organic&th=1

Freeze Dried Berries

Blueberries: https://smile.amazon.com/gp/product/B019P50NSE/ref=ppx _yo_dt_b_asin_title_o01__o00_s00?ie=UTF8&th=1

Berry selection: https://smile.amazon.com/s?k=freeze+dried+berries &ref=is_s

Freeze-dried pomegranate: https://smile.amazon.com/Karens-Naturals-Pomegranate-Freeze-Dried-Preservatives/dp/B00ARKRO2A/ref= mp_s_a_1_3?crid=3MA9OPXT3X2FJ&keywords=pomegranate+seeds +for+eating&qid=1550552220&s=gateway&sprefix=pomegranate+se eds&sr=8-3

Freeze-dried acai powder: https://smile.amazon.com/Organic-ACAI-Powder-Freeze-Dried-Antioxidant/dp/B01BCCYJHE/ref=mp_s_a_1_4? crid=2VKNPLOWQ5YPQ&keywords=acai+seeds&qid=1550553286&s= gateway&sprefix=acai+seeds&sr=8-4

Kefir Starter for Milk (Dairy or Non-Dairy): https://www.amazon.com /Yogourmet-Freeze-Dried-Kefir-Starter/dp/B000LKXRWC/ ref=sr_1_1?ie=UTF8&qid=1550511259&sr=8-1&keywords= yogourmet+kefir+starter

Water Kefir: https://smile.amazon.com/Grains-Cultures-Health-Organic -Gluten/dp/B002ZIDELM/ref=sr_1_3_a_it?ie=UTF8&qid=1550681874 &sr=8-3&keywords=Real+kefir+water

Whole Pumpkin Seed Kernels: https://smile.amazon.com/Lightly-Salted-Whole-Pumpkin-Shell/dp/B00EOVIO5O

Fresh Food

Farmers' Markets by zip code: https://localfarmersmarket.us/

Locavore (phone app): https://apps.apple.com/us/app/locavore/id306140158

Food Literacy

Slow Food USA: https://www.slowfoodusa.org/blog-post/why-slow-food-policy-matters-the-2018-farm-bill

International Scientific Association for Probiotics and Prebiotics (microbiome education): https://isappscience.org/

Recipe Websites

Vegetarian Meal Ideas: https://vegmealideas.com/

Eating Well: http://www.eatingwell.com/

Manjulas Kitchen: https://www.manjulaskitchen.com/

Vegetable Gardening

The Spruce: https://www.thespruce.com/growing-vegetables-a-to-z-1403435

Plants

Neem Tree Farms (Neem, Moringa, Tulsi, Aloe Plants): https://neem-treefarms.com/

Seeds for Your Vegetable Garden

Johnny's Selected Seeds: https://www.johnnyseeds.com/

Kitazawa Seed Company: https://www.kitazawaseed.com/

Seed Saver Exchange: https://www.seedsavers.org/

Row 7 Seeds https://www.row7seeds.com/

Organic Produce Delivered to Your Door

Amazon Prime Now (phone app): https://primenow.amazon.com/onboard?forceOnboard=1&sourceUrl=%2Fhome

Farm Fresh To You: http://www.farmfreshtoyou.com/

Local Harvest: https://www.localharvest.org/vista-ca

Instacart (phone app): https://shoppers.instacart.com/apps

Thrive Market (phone app): https://thrivemarket.com/get-the-app

Organic Produce Inventory

Veggie Seasons (phone app): https://apps.apple.com/us/app/veggie-seasons/id1450855435

Shopping for Healthy Food

Eat Wild: http://eatwild.com/products/index.html

Real Milk: https://www.realmilk.com/

Chapter 4: Move Your Body

Movement

Gokhale Method for pain-free back: https://gokhalemethod.com/

Yoga Websites and Apps

Daily Yoga: https://www.dailyyoga.com/

Daily Yoga app: https://apps.apple.com/us/app/daily-yoga-workout-fitness/id545849922

Do Yoga With Me: https://www.doyogawithme.com/

Gaiam, Yoga Studio app: https://www.gaiam.com/blogs/discover/yoga-studio-by-gaiam-app

Health: https://www.health.com/

Yoga Basics: https://yogabasics.com/

Yoga YouTube Videos

You will find a few useful pointers for yoga asanas in these YouTube videos. However, a group or individual lesson with a competent yoga teacher is advisable: https://youtu.be/v7AYKMP6rOE and https://youtu.be/lfwsGu6seCA

Exercise Aids and Gadgets

All Purpose Non-Slip Exercise Yoga Mat with Carrying Strap: https://smile.amazon.com/BalanceFrom-Purpose-Non-Slip-Exercise-Carrying/dp/B01IZDFWY2/ref=mp_s_a_1_5?crid=2CBBZBY4ZPJL8&keywords=yoga+mat&qid=1550261158&s=gateway&sprefix=yoga+m&sr=8-5

Folding Trampoline (36 inch): https://smile.amazon.com/Stamina-Trampoline-Workouts-Included-Supports/dp/B000JC2ZHA/ref=mp_s_a_1_5?crid=32B9XW2OMM5JE&hasWorkingJavascript=1&keywords=trampoline&qid=1550260011&s=gateway&sprefix=trampoline&sr=8-5

Lumbar Support Back Cushion for lower back pain relief: https://smile.amazon.com/LoveHome-Balanced-Firmness-Designed-Computer/dp/B00D5J7SL2/ref=mp_s_a_1_28?crid=23AGYHHAKP3M1&keywords=posture+back+support&qid=1550260338&s=gateway&sprefix=posture+back&sr=8-28

Ball Chair/Exercise Yoga Ball for improved balance, back pain relief, core strength, and posture: https://smile.amazon.com/Trideer-Ball-Chair-Stability-Resistance/dp/B07CLYLRXT/ref=mp_s_a_1_38?crid=2177F3IDHHU23&keywords=inflatable+chair&qid=15502698&s=gateway&sprefix=inflatable+chair&sr=8-38

Jump Rope, adjustable with comfortable handles: https://smile.amazon.com/Limm-All-Purpose-Jump-Rope/dp/B00VOCG44O/ref=mp_s

_a_1_6?crid=2MBUV6D68MMHK&keywords=jump%2Brope&qid=1550260074&s=gateway&sprefix=jump%2Brope&sr=8-6&th=1&psc=1

Chapter 5: Restore Yourself

Fun with Cooking

Kids Cook Real Food: https://kidscookrealfood.com

Sleeping Aids and Gadgets

Cleveland Clinic: Go! To Sleep Online Program: https://shop.clevelandclinicwellness.com/collections/online-programs/products/go-to-sleep-online

Natural Silk Sleep Mask: https://www.amazon.com/ALASKA-BEAR-Natural-blindfold-super-smooth/dp/B00S5Q826U/ref=mp_s_a_1_7?crid=IOVU28GUQVV4&keywords=nidra+deep+rest+sleep+mask&qid=1550509784&s=gateway&sprefix=nidra+&sr=8-7

Sleep Cycle app: https://www.sleepcycle.com/

SleepScore Labs app: https://shop.sleepscore.com/pages/apps

Volunteering Programs

AARP Foundation Experience Corps https://www.aarp.org/experience-corps/

Encore: https://encore.org/

Gen2Gen: https://generationtogeneration.org/about-us/

Chapter 6: Practice Mindfulness

Online Resources for Meditation Practices

Self-Realization Fellowship: https://yogananda.org/a-beginners-meditation

Chapter 7: Build Your Health Team

For an explanation of NNT: https://www.thennt.com/thennt-explained/)

For current recommendations on mammograms: https://www.cdc.gov/cancer/breast/pdf/breastcancerscreeningguidelines.pdf.)

Wellness Education

Body Ecology: https://bodyecology.com/

Frank Lipman, M.D.: https://drfranklipman.com/

Cleveland Clinic, Stress Free Now Online Clinic: https://shop.clevelandclinicwellness.com/collections/online-programs/products/stress-free-now-online-program

Where to Find Holistic Doctors and Healers

American Association of Naturopathic Physicians: https://naturopathic.org/

American College for Advancement in Medicine: https://www.acam.org/default.aspx

Health Insurers and Providers websites

Institute of Functional Medicine: https://www.ifm.org/

Paleo Physicians Network: http://www.paleophysiciansnetwork.com/

Re-Find Health: https://re-findhealth.com/

For the Cost-Sharing Insurance Model in a Healthy Empowered Community

Knew Health: https://knewhealth.com/

Other Health Resources

Canadian Deprescribing Network: https://www.deprescribingnetwork.ca/canadian-deprescribing-network/?smid=nytcore-ios-shares

Health Advocate

AARP Advocacy: https://www.aarp.org/politics-society/advocacy/

Chapter 8: Homemade Hygiene Products

DIY Beauty Regimen

Wellness Mama: https://wellnessmama.com/

Glass Bottle Sprayer for Deodorant: https://www.amazon.com/Empty-Amber-Glass-Bottles-Labels/dp/B01G98Y1BA/ref=mp_s_a_1_3?crid=2VWVU1GBNHH8A&keywords=bottle+sprayer&qid=1550509911&s=gateway&sprefix=bottle+spra&sr=8-3

Chapter 9: Guidelines for Healthy Meals

Cooking Aids and Gadgets

Two-Tier Lazy Susan for spice rack: https://smile.amazon.com/Lipper-International-8302-Kitchen-Turntable/dp/B001D33RWQ

Cast Iron Mini Skillet 3.5 Inch: https://smile.amazon.com/Lodge-Skillet-Miniature-Individual-Desserts/dp/B000LXA9YI/ref=mp_s_a_1_17?keywords=small+pan+one+egg&qid=1550294836&s=gateway&sr=8-17

Electric Spice and Coffee Grinder: https://smile.amazon.com/KRUPS-Electric-Coffee-Grinder-Stainless/dp/B00004SPEU/ref=mp_s_a_1_3?crid=2RRVFRYU17369&keywords=coffee+grinder&qid=1550259550&s=gateway&sprefix=coffee&sr=8-3

Handheld Garlic peeler: https://smile.amazon.com/OXO-Silicone-Garlic-Stay-Clean-Storage/dp/B0002YTFV4

Handheld Vegetable Slicer/Spiralizer for salad making: https://smile.amazon.com/Vegetable-XBrands-Different-Multi-Function-Shredded/dp/B07JM6YBX6

Instant Pot, 7 in 1 programmable pressure cooker: https://instantpot.com/ and https://www.amazon.com/dp/B00FLYWNYQ?aaxitk=Pr4wPhGceX6i7uUSLaG3ZA&pd_rd_i=B00FLYWNYQ&pf_rd_p=3ff6092e-8451-438b-8278-7e94064b4d42&hsa_cr_id=9377393360901&sb-ci-n=productDescription&sb-ci-v=Instant%20Pot%20DUO60%206%20Qt%207-in-1%20Multi-Use%20Programmable%20Pressure%20Cooker%2C%20Slow%20Cooker%2C%20Rice%20Cooker%2C%20Steamer%2C%20Saut%C3%A9%2C%20Yogurt%20Maker%20and%20Warmer

Magnetic Dry Erase Weekly Planner for Fridge: https://www.amazon.com/Holiday-Gift-Magnetic-Whiteboard-60876668980/dp/B01J23JSE4/ref=sr_1_3?ie=UTF8&qid=1550511694&sr=8-3&keywords=magnetic+dry+erase+board+for+refrigerator

Non-contact Digital Laser Infrared Thermometer Temperature Gun: https://smile.amazon.com/Etekcity-Lasergrip-774-Non-contact-Thermometer/dp/B00837ZGRY/ref=mp_s_a_1_15?crid=13RTJ0A4TW9LT&keywords=food+thermometer&qid=1550295533&s=gateway&sprefix=food+thermo&sr=8-15

Spice Jars Bottles - 14 (4 oz.): https://smile.amazon.com/Spice-Jars-Bottles-Containers-Chalkboard/dp/B07193N71J/ref=mp_s_a_1_15?crid=2UL7U79SBCL3G&keywords=rectangular+spice+rack&qid=1550258971&s=gateway&sprefix=rectangular+spice+&sr=8-15

Stainless Steel Colander Sets Wire Filter Mesh for Sprouting: https://smile.amazon.com/CHICHIC-Stainless-Strainers-Colander-Vegetable/dp/B018LBXJYI/ref=mp_s_a_1_6?keywords=strainer&qid=1550259195&s=gateway&sr=8-6

Sprouting Strainer Lid for Wide Mouth Mason Jars: https://smile.amazon.com/Sprouting-Resistant-Stainless-Strainer-Canning/dp/B07H81Q4HT/ref=mp_s_a_1_8?keywords=strainer+with+lid&qid=1550259307&s=gateway&sr=8-8

Stainless Steel Tea Infuser: https://smile.amazon.com/Senbowe-Stainless-Infuser-Strainer-Steeper/dp/B07MM57TLX/ref=mp_s_a_1_12?crid=1MW70TJHSZPS9&keywords=strainer+tea+infuser&qid=1550259393&s=gateway&sprefix=strainer+tea+&sr=8-12

Acknowledgments

First, I thank my cardiologist, Erminia Guarneri, for shepherding me to health and for writing the foreword to this book. I bow to the ordering principle of universe to bring the ancient Vedic wisdom of Ayurveda and the recent paradigm-shifting discoveries in health sciences together to empower us with the wisdom that lifestyle primarily governs and regulates our health, and averts all diseases.

In the same spirit, this book is a creative process larger than the author alone. I remember the face of an elderly lady in my class at Oasis who chastised me and asked, "When are you going to write a book so I don't have to take these copious notes?" Breck Allen, Neha Patel, Ranjan Varma Sunil Arora, Suresh Ramaswamy, and Tom Dwyer, constantly encouraged me and gave me confidence in completing this task. They envisioned it as a finished product before I could.

Upon inception, my developmental editor, Cherie Kephart has been the key architect of this book ever since I first shared the outline with her. She brought the whole editing/publishing team together as well, which enabled this book to become a reality. If I am the composer, Cherie is the maestro conductor. Playing a symphonic role is my copy editor, Janet F. Williams, who fine-tuned the writing, made sense of these pages, and cleaned up the music. She has my sincere gratitude.

Special thanks to my Amitabh Divakar for creating a cover design that embues humility and grace while emphasizing the innate essence of vitality in all of us. Thank you also to Nawal Singh for his illustrations and Amit Dey for composition, for you both conveyed my words in an extraordinary way.

My thanks to those who shared their favorite recipes: Akhilesh Maewal, Amitabh Divakar, Binita Sinha, Jaishree Bhushan, Manjula Jain, Meena Sinha, and Veena Verma.

Thanks to the early readers of my book: Breck Allen, John Salatti, and Miguel Watley. They have all sharpened, brightened, and enhanced this book.

For everyone involved in this project, thank you for your expertise and confidence in me. However, any errors or shortcomings in this book are completely mine.

Last, but by no means least, I am thankful to my ashramites here at the Hidden Valley Ashram. They all helped me heal and lead a healthy lifestyle in body, mind, and spirit so this book became possible.

It is with a deep sense of gratitude and humility, and on behalf of all above, I offer this book to my readers. It is my prayer that this book is helpful to my readers, and their friends and loved ones in leading a healthy life.

About the Author

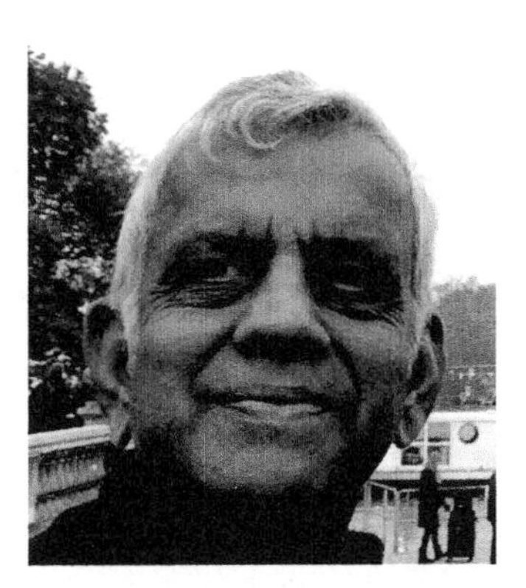

Ravi Sahay is an author, inspirational speaker, and educator. As an adjunct faculty member at the College of Humanities and Sciences at the University of Phoenix, San Diego, Ravi was given the Faculty Scholar Award for his first book, *My Health is Your Wealth*. In that very personal, but universally significant account, Ravi describes his own battle with many health challenges including a heart attack, congestive heart failure, urinary tract infections, sinusitis, systemic candida, and chronic eczema. The book shares his triumph over all of these ailments through the combination of integrative medicine and a lifestyle dedicated to wellness.

Having such a keen interest in the economics of healthcare and the future of our well-being, Ravi was inspired to write his second book, *May You BE Healthy: Well-being for Pennies a Day*. Ravi is passionate about empowering others with what he has discovered as essential knowledge to making the best decisions about our health.

Connect with Ravi at: RaviSahay.com

More Books by Ravi Sahay

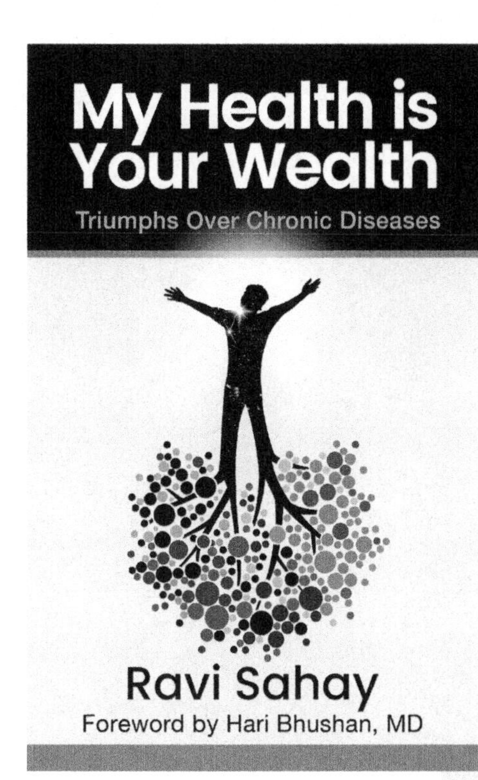

"Ravi has done an excellent job of stepping out of the box and looking at health and wellness through a new perspective."

~ Mimi Guarneri, MD, FACC

"Ravi Sahay's infinite persistence in seeking a cure for his many ailments will be inspirational for fellow afflicted sufferers. The wisdom and experience of integrated holistic treatment approaches, including Ayurveda, nutrition, and diet has enabled Mr. Sahay to produce an eloquent and coherent plea for a more effective, rational, and cost-effective medical system."

~ Sandra Goodman, Ph.D., Editor and Director,
Positive Health Publications Ltd.

"Ravi, your book is excellent--a good introduction in natural health."

~ Frank Cuny, Executive Director,
California Citizens for Health Freedom

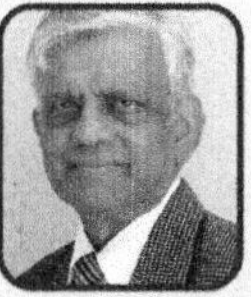

RAVI SAHAY exemplifies the power of lifestyle changes by using an integrative (holistic) approach in healing and prevention for chronic conditions. Ravi shares the wisdom in his books, ***May You BE Healthy: Well-being for Pennies a Day***, and ***My Health is Your Wealth: Triumphs Over Chronic Diseases.*** Ancient Indian Ayurvedic wisdom and the recent rediscovery of the microbiome empowered him on this vigorous journey.

Ravi immigrated to the United States from India in 1971 with an Electrical Engineering degree; earned two master's degrees in EE and business, and rose up the corporate ladder. Along the way his health started to fail. In mid-life, Ravi struggled with several chronic diseases including heart disease, high blood pressure, and skin, gum, sinus and fatigue problems. After his heart attack in 2003, Ravi enrolled in Dean Ornish's Heart Healthy program where Mimi Guarneri, MD became his Integrative Medicine cardiologist. Dr. Guarneri shepherded Ravi to full recovery. She has written the foreword and testimonial to his books. Ravi taught economics and math at the University of Phoenix, San Diego campus, and received a scholarly award for ***My Health is Your Wealth.*** Ravi lives in San Diego and speaks and writes on ways to reduce our healthcare costs and improve our well-being.

ravisahay.com

Made in the USA
Middletown, DE
19 February 2021

34042277R00119